Histologic Preparations

Common Problems and Their Solutions

Richard W. Brown, MD
Editor

Developed by the
College of American Pathologists

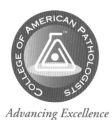

Advancing Excellence

In conjunction with the
National Society for Histotechnology

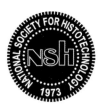

Library of Congress Control Number: 2009924500
ISBN: 978-0-930304-95-9
Printed in the USA

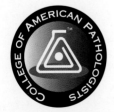

Advancing Excellence

College of American Pathologists
325 Waukegan Road
Northfield, Illinois 60093
800-323-4040

Contributors

Richard W. Brown, MD
Memorial Hermann Healthcare System
Houston, Texas

Freida L. Carson, PhD, HT(ASCP)
Baylor University Medical Center (Retired)
Dallas, Texas

Vinnie Della Speranza, MS, HTL(ASCP)HT
Medical University of South Carolina
Charleston, South Carolina

Sue E. Lewis, HTL(ASCP)QIHC
University of Iowa Hospitals and Clinics
Iowa City, Iowa

Robert L. Lott, HTL(ASCP)
Trinity Medical Center / LabFirst
Birmingham, Alabama

Lena T. Spencer, MA, HTL(ASCP)QIHC
Norton Healthcare
Louisville, Kentucky

Janet Tunnicliffe, MLT ART
Fraser Health Authority, Laboratory
Royal Columbian Hospital
New Westminster, BC, Canada

Contents

Preface

Histologic Preparations: Common Problems and Their Solutions is an extension of the National Society for Histotechnology / College of American Pathologists (NSH / CAP) HistoQIP program, the first program in the United States through which laboratories can obtain an objective evaluation of quality for the histologic sections, special stains, and immunohistochemical preparations they prepare. From the inception of this program in 2003, it was the intention of the sponsoring CAP / NSH Histotechnology Resource Committee to provide participating laboratories with meaningful feedback regarding the problems noted in their slides. The educational critiques for this program typically include information regarding the common causes of problems encountered and ways in which they may be prevented.

Histologic Preparations represents a greatly expanded version of these critiques. Each chapter is organized similarly. After a brief presentation of the technique or stain, including the underlying biochemistry where applicable, there is a list of common problems encountered by laboratories using that stain or technique and a number of possible solutions. The numerous illustrations in this text include examples of excellent quality preparations and the problems that can occur. Many are derived from slides received in the HistoQIP program.

Histologic Preparations is intended to serve as a reference for histotechnology students and histotechnicians at the bench, pathology residents, and perhaps most importantly, the pathologists serving as medical directors of histology laboratories, who are regularly called upon to provide not only an assessment of slide quality but also the first line of problem identification and troubleshooting.

Richard W. Brown, MD, FCAP

Fixation and Processing

Freida L. Carson

Fixation

Fixation is the single most influential factor in the long sequence of steps between procurement of the specimen and coverslipping the stained slide; nearly any other step can be reversed to ameliorate a problem. Tissues can be reverse-processed and then reprocessed if a mistake or breakdown occurs in tissue processing. Most stains can be removed and reapplied to correct problems with intensity or specificity. Bubbles under the coverslip can be removed simply by removing and resetting the coverslip. In sharp contrast to these examples, errors in fixation are permanent. On the positive side, properly fixed tissue is nearly impervious to abuse during tissue processing and slide preparation. Understanding the role and mechanism of fixation is crucial to producing quality slides and interpreting artifacts. Important aspects can be grouped under four rules.

Rule #1 is that fixatives denature macromolecules; ie, fixation changes the shape of large molecules. This rule is the basis for the varied functions of fixation and why fixed specimens look the way they do under the microscope. Thus:

a. Fixation kills cells because denatured molecules can no longer engage in life-supporting chemical reactions.

b. Fixation prevents autolysis because biological activity of the specimen's enzymes is destroyed as their shape is altered.

c. Fixation prevents microbial attack because substrates are no longer recognizable in their new conformation.

d. Fixation firms the tissue (making it easier to gross and to section) because denatured molecules form new intramolecular and intermolecular bonds.

e. Fixation changes the tissue's receptivity to stains and histochemical procedures. In most cases the influence is positive because procedures have been optimized to work with fixed tissue, but prominent negative examples exist (eg, masking of antigenic sites necessary for immunohistochemical staining).

Rule #2 is that different fixatives produce their own morphological patterns. That is an objective fact that does not imply good or bad. Whether we like what we see is a subjective matter predominantly based on our individual training. Many chemicals act as fixatives in that they denature macromolecules, but few produce "acceptable" results because each creates its own unique pattern of changes visible at the level of the light microscope. We speak of "formaldehyde patterns" (implying "good") versus "alcohol patterns" ("bad") in describing how a specimen appears under the microscope. Some observers give high preference to mercuric fixatives over neutral buffered formalin (NBF) for lymphoid tissues, and picric acid for gastric biopsies, because of the extra-sharp images they produce. Defining "good" fixation, then, is difficult because of varying personal preferences. However, there are well-documented and accepted minimum staining criteria that specify well-defined nuclear patterns, epithelial cell membranes, and cytoplasmic staining exhibited by well-fixed tissues.[1,2]

Rule #3 is that fixation is a chemical reaction that is not instantaneous. Its rate is dependent upon the chemical nature of the fixative solution and its temperature. Closely correlated with this is Rule #4, which says that a fixative must be present for any reaction to occur. This self-evident notion is so frequently ignored that it warrants discussion. Raw specimens are not freely porous objects. Fluids of any sort take time to diffuse into the mass. If there are numerous intercellular channels, as in lymph nodes, movement is faster than if cells are tightly adherent to one another, but penetration still is not instantaneous. Most specimens present membrane barriers that must be crossed each time the fluid moves into the next cell. Because membranes have fatty interiors, aqueous fixatives penetrate poorly. Alcoholic versions of common fixatives (alcoholic formalin, alcoholic zinc formalin, and alcoholic glyoxal) are able to penetrate much faster.

In most cases fixation increases permeability, but some fixing agents (eg, mercuric salts) create such tight

Table 1.1. Fixation/Processing Errors on the 2003-2004 HQIP H&E Challenges

Tissue H&E	% Fixation Delayed	% Fixation Incomplete	% Excessive Dehydration	% Poor Processing	% Cell Shrinkage	% Formalin or Mercury Pigment	% Nuclear Bubbling	% Excessive Decalcification	% Poor Section Orientation
Breast	2	14	1	9	0	2	9	NA	0
Skin	0	10	1	5	0	1	7	NA	2
Lymph Node	7	30	5	7	3	3	0	NA	0
Lung	7	11	2	3	2	6	5	NA	0
Uterus	11	19	0	3	1	1	27	NA	0
Colon	15	20	0	3	2	1	8	NA	2
Bone Marrow	5	16	1	11	2	1	3	8	0
Liver	8	12	5	6	1	0	8	NA	0
Average	**7**	**17**	**2**	**8**	**1**	**2**	**8**	**NA**	**0.5**

intermolecular bonds that diffusion may be impeded, and the fixative cannot penetrate all the way into the specimen. While alcoholic solutions of aldehyde fixatives do not seem to affect permeability adversely, plain alcohol used for dehydration certainly does.

Rules #3 and #4 dictate that adequate time be given for the fixation process (penetration + chemical reaction). Beyond that, no physical encumbrances should be introduced during the handling of specimen. Squeezing with forceps introduces localized artifacts because penetration is hindered at the sites of tissue damage. More commonly, forcing oversized chunks of tissue into a cassette inhibits or prevents penetration by any fluid and may render processing an exercise in futility. The tissue will remain unfixed, processing fluids will not dehydrate or clear, and the block will not section. If such a disaster is then trimmed thinner and reprocessed, sections may be possible, but the tissue will be rotten. There is no excuse for overly thick specimens.

Processing

If tissue is completely fixed, processing problems are less likely to occur. However, today's laboratory practices requiring ever faster turnaround times can result in incompletely fixed specimens, so proper processing is imperative to minimize the overall detrimental effect. The most common problems in processing are caused by processing both biopsy and large tissue specimens simultaneously on the same processing program. This leads to overprocessing and excessive dehydration of the biopsy tissues and/or underprocessing and incomplete dehydration of the larger specimens. These tissues should be processed separately and on different schedules. As stated in the previous section under "Fixation," tissues must be cut as thin as possible, with the optimum thickness being no more than 3 mm, or about the thickness of a nickel. A problem that has been encountered frequently within the last decade or so is one that leads to very poor staining of the nucleus. In the United States this problem is referred to as smudginess or blue halo effect, and in the United Kingdom as "nuclear meltdown." This is most often caused by incomplete dehydration prior to clearing, but using too much heat on the processor will also cause this same poor staining pattern.

Heat should be used only for the paraffin, and that should be at a temperature just above the melting point of the paraffin. These problems will be discussed more completely in the problem-solving section of this chapter. The most common fixation and processing problems on the 2003–2004 National Society for Histotechnology/College of American Pathologists (NSH/CAP) HistoQIP (HQIP) program hematoxylin and eosin (H&E) challenges are shown in Table 1.1. Percentages have been rounded to the nearest whole percent. The special stain challenges are not included because the problems are not always as apparent on special stains.

What Should Be Seen in a Well-Fixed, Well-Processed Specimen Stained With Hematoxylin and Eosin

- Nuclei should show a variety of chromatin patterns, with a crisp blue nuclear membrane. There should not be any nuclear bubbling, smudginess, or fading.
- The cell cytoplasm should be well preserved and should stain well with eosin.
- There should not be any artifactual spaces between the individual cells.
- There should not be any cell shrinkage.

A well-fixed and well-processed section of small intestine is demonstrated in Figure 1.1.[3] The nuclei show a variety of chromatin patterns, with crisp nuclear membranes. There is no cell shrinkage; the cell membranes are sharply defined, and the mucin droplets in the goblet cells and the brush border of the epithelium are also well preserved. This tissue was fixed for 7 hours in zinc-formalin.

Excellent fixation and processing of lymphoid tissue is illustrated in Figure 1.2. There is excellent nuclear detail in the germinal center, with eosinophilic nucleoli seen in several nuclei. Nuclei with a variety of chromatin patterns can be seen, and no artifactual spaces are seen around the lymphocytes. This tissue was received in neutral buffered formalin early in the morning, sectioned, put into cassettes, and fixed until 6:00 pm, when it was put on the processor on an overnight schedule. The first three stations on the processor are alcoholic formalin.

A number of the most common fixation and processing problems are discussed and demonstrated in the following pages. It should be noted that in many instances fixation and processing problems have multiple and varied outcomes, so it is not always possible to correlate one problem with only one solution.

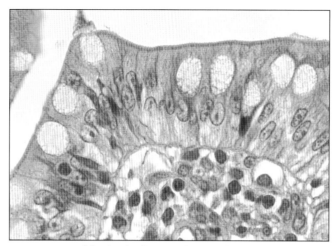

Figure 1.1. A well-fixed and well-processed section of small intestine is demonstrated in this image. A variety of chromatin patterns can be seen in the nuclei, and the nuclear membranes are crisp and sharply defined. No cell shrinkage is noted.

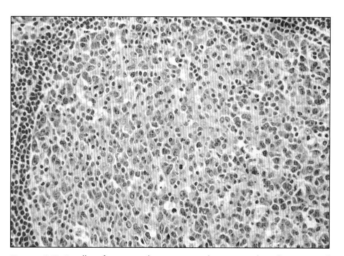

Figure 1.2. Excellent fixation and processing is demonstrated on this section of lymphoid tissue. The nuclear detail is excellent in the germinal center, with a variety of chromatin patterns seen. Eosinophilic nucleoli can be seen in several nuclei.

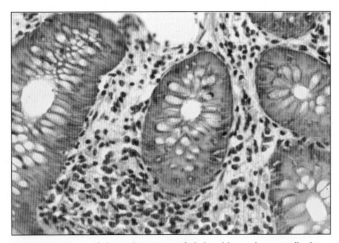

Figure 1.3. Some of the nuclei are very faded and have almost totally disappeared in this section of intestine, while others are very pyknotic. This is a manifestation of early autolysis or delayed fixation.[3]

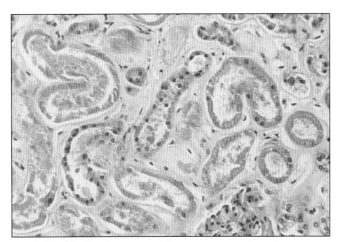

Figure 1.4. The effects of mild autolysis can be seen in this section of kidney. No nuclei remain in some of the tubules.

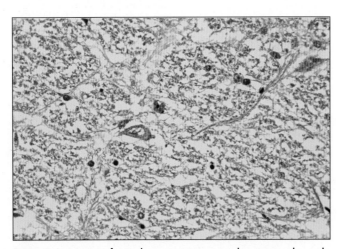

Figure 1.5. A section of central nervous system tissue demonstrates the results of delayed fixation, with marked disruption of the normal morphology.

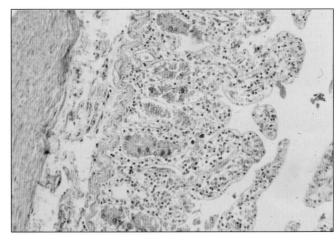

Figure 1.6. Except for the crypts, the epithelial layer has totally disappeared in this very autolysed section of small intestine. This is typical of delayed fixation of autopsy tissues, and sections of this type should not be used as control tissue.

Problems Encountered With Fixation and Processing

PROBLEM: Fixation Delayed

APPEARANCE: Nuclei may show a loss of chromatin, blue halo, fading, or complete disappearance (Figures 1.3 and 1.4). There may be cell shrinkage, disruption of the cytoplasm, and artifactual spaces around cells (Figure 1.5). If the delay is prolonged, some cells may completely disappear, such as the epithelial cells in intestinal specimens obtained at autopsy (Figure 1.6).

CAUSES:

- Specimens are obtained long after the blood supply has been compromised (eg, autopsy).
- The specimen is not opened so that fixative can come in contact with all surfaces (eg, uterus, small intestine, colon).
- The specimen is not thinly cut so that fixatives can penetrate more easily (eg, spleen, breast, organ resections, large tumors).
- Inadequate volume of fixative relative to the amount of tissue (20:1 minimum).

SOLUTIONS:

- Place specimens in fixative as soon as possible after the blood supply has been interrupted.
- Open specimens wherever possible. Gastrointestinal specimens should be opened, pinned to a cork or paraffin wax board, and placed in fixative. Uterus specimens should also be opened and placed in fixative. Lungs can be inflated with fixative by gravity flow.
- Slice specimens, such as spleen, breast, kidney, any organ resection, or large tumor, into thin slices and place in fixative.

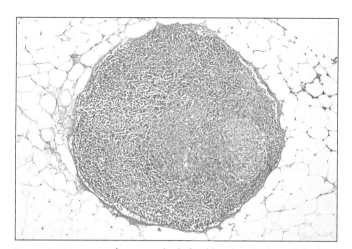

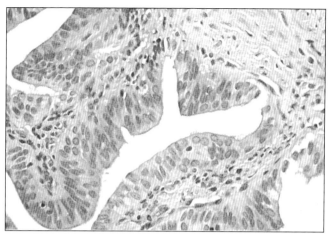

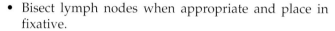

Figure 1.7. A section of an incompletely fixed lymph node shows slight disintegration in the water bath due to incomplete fixation. This node is completely surrounded by fat and was not bisected; thus the fixative had a difficult time penetrating.

Figure 1.8. A section of fallopian tube demonstrates "smudgy" or "muddy" nuclei that result from incomplete fixation. The nuclear chromatin patterns would be much more apparent after a longer period of fixation.

- Bisect lymph nodes when appropriate and place in fixative.
- Place formalin container for holding cassettes on stir plates, and provide agitation to enhance the fixation and penetration process.
- Ensure that the volume of fixative is 15 to 20 times that of the tissue.
- Sort cassettes by specimen thickness and size for appropriate processing schedule.

PROBLEM: Fixation Incomplete

APPEARANCE: Nuclei may be muddy, or smudgy. Tissue components can separate easily on the flotation bath during microtomy. Tissue morphology is not well maintained (Figures 1.7, 1.8, and 1.9).

CAUSES:
- Tissue sections not allowed enough time in fixative.
- Inadequate amount of fixative relative to tissue volume.
- Sections grossed too thick for good penetration.
- Formalin solution is depleted.

SOLUTIONS:
- Ensure that enough time is allowed for good fixation (see "Comments").
- Ensure that the fixative volume is 15 to 20 times the tissue volume.
- Ensure that the grossed sections are thin, preferably no more than 3 mm thick.
- Change formalin solutions frequently throughout the process to prevent depletion.

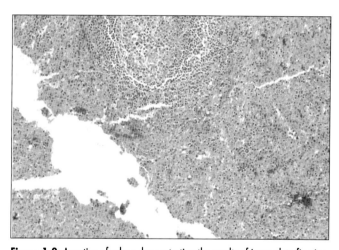

Figure 1.9. A section of spleen demonstrating the results of incomplete fixation. There is a large crack that occurred during flotation on the water bath due to the incomplete fixation. The white pulp also shows the poor cell adhesion due to the inadequate fixation. This problem will not occur with well-fixed tissue.

COMMENTS: Well-grossed sections of routine tissue should be fixed at least 8 to 12 hours to ensure at least adequate fixation; however, various authorities have stated that anywhere from 48 hours to 1 week is necessary for complete fixation. In a carefully controlled study, Dapson[3] found that artifact-free specimens could be produced with neutral buffered formalin fixation only if they were fixed a minimum of 30 to 40 hours, and that profound artifacts were apparent after 7 hours of fixative exposure. The use of alcoholic formalin on the tissue processor will help this somewhat, but enough exposure time is still needed between the tissue and the fixative solution. Excellent sections can be obtained after only 7 hours fixation in zinc formalin (see Figure 1.1).[3] Thin sections are critical in all instances for good fixation.

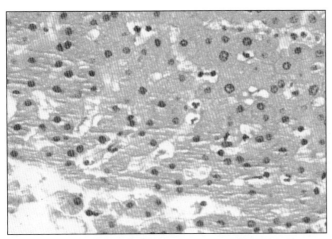

Figure 1.10. A liver biopsy showing the effects of over-dehydration. This artifact (chatter) is especially apparent at the edge of the tissue. This tissue also shows the effects of incomplete fixation, where cells present a homogenous appearance, with no nuclear detail and poorly stained hepatocyte cytoplasm.

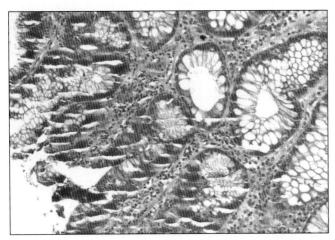

Figure 1.11. Gastrointestinal biopsy showing the effects of over-dehydration, with microchatter seen at the edge of the tissue. This section is also too thick.

PROBLEM: Tissue Excessively Dehydrated

APPEARANCE: Microchatter is most commonly seen at the edges of the tissue, especially biopsy specimens. Hairline cracks may also be seen in the tissue (Figures 1.10 and 1.11).

CAUSES:

- Too much time is allowed in the dehydrating solutions.
- Molecularly bound water is removed as well as the free water.

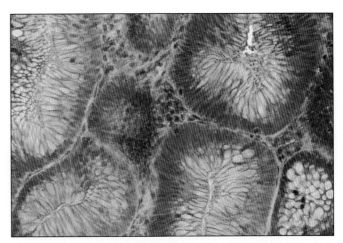

Figure 1.12. A gastrointestinal biopsy showing a marked lack of clarity and cellular detail. This is attributed to incomplete dehydration in the processor.

- Processing biopsy tissues on the same schedule as larger specimens.
- Processing biopsy tissues on a schedule that is too long.

SOLUTIONS:

- Decrease time in dehydrating solutions.
- Use a shorter processing schedule for biopsy tissues.
- Process biopsy tissues separately from large specimens.

PROBLEM: Tissue Poorly Processed

APPEARANCE: The section may appear cloudy, with the nuclei varying in staining properties. There is no chromatin definition in the nuclei, and some nuclei may appear very "washed out" (Figures 1.12 and 1.13).

CAUSES:

- Residual water remaining in tissues when they are placed in clearing agent.
- Fixative left in tissues when placed in clearing agent.
- Incomplete paraffin infiltration.
- Too much clearing agent in paraffin.
- Too much heat during processing.

SOLUTIONS:

- Ensure that the last alcohols are anhydrous.
- Ensure that fixative and alcohol droplets are not condensing on the processor chamber lid and then dropping into the processing chamber.

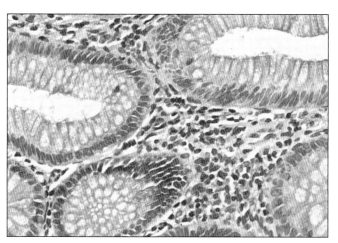

Figure 1.13. The washed out nuclei in this section are due to too much heat applied during processing. (Image courtesy of Richard Dapson.)

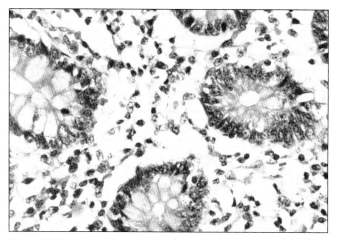

Figure 1.14. A section of gastrointestinal tract that demonstrates cell shrinkage as a result of inadequate fixation. (Image courtesy of Richard Dapson.)

- Have the processor checked for malfunctioning valves, sealant rings, or washers.
- Ensure that paraffin is changed on a regular schedule to prevent carryover or contamination from fixation and/or processing reagents.
- Ensure that all solution residues are completely cleaned from the retort (follow manufacturer's guidelines for periodic maintenance such as a warm water flush).
- Ensure that all processing solutions are kept at the lowest temperature possible; only paraffin should have heat applied.

COMMENTS: This artifact sometimes seems to come and go with no apparent reason. Although the cause of sections with this appearance has been attributed to several different things, including bad formaldehyde solutions, it is most often caused by incomplete dehydration of the tissue before the clearing step in processing, or condensation of the fixative on the processor lid followed by contamination of the succeeding reagents.[4] This problem is worse on small tissues, such as skin, endometrium, and gastrointestinal biopsies. It has been reported that this artifact can be partially reversed in tissues by heating with the BioGenex antigen retrieval solution,[5] or by boiling sections in any solution designed for heat induced epitope retrieval (HIER) or in just water.

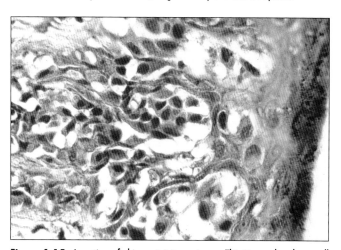

Figure 1.15. A section of skin containing a tumor. This tissue also shows cell shrinkage.

PROBLEM: Cell Shrinkage

APPEARANCE: Cells are shrunken and there are a lot of artifactual spaces around the cells. The nuclei may also appear pyknotic (Figures 1.14 and 1.15).

CAUSES:
- Inadequate fixation followed by excessive dehydration.
- Drying before submersion in fixative.

SOLUTIONS:
- Ensure adequate fixation before beginning processing.
- Ensure that specimens do not dry prior to immersion in fixative.

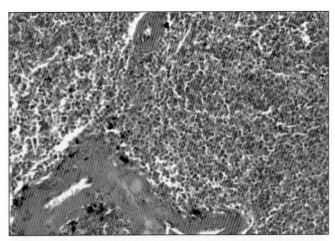

Figure 1.16. A section of spleen containing marked formalin pigment. This section is also not well fixed or well stained.

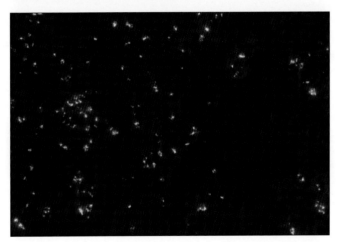

Figure 1.17. A section containing formalin pigment examined with polarization. This is a good method of checking for the presence of formalin pigment when it is not obvious on H&E-stained sections.

PROBLEM: Formalin or Mercury Pigment

APPEARANCE: Brown to black pigments in the tissue; formalin pigment is most prevalent in bloody tissues. These pigments usually lie on top of the cells, although rarely formalin pigment can occur within cells (Figures 1.16, 1.17, and 1.18).

CAUSES:

- Formalin solution has a pH below 5.5.
- Tissue is very bloody.
- Tissue has not been treated to remove mercury pigment.

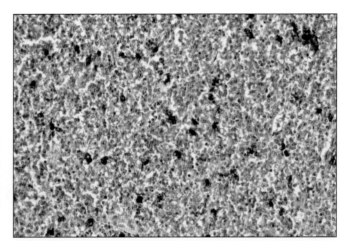

Figure 1.18. A section of spleen containing mercury pigment. This pigment is usually blacker, and the pigment deposition is larger than with formalin. Also, staining is usually not optimal when the pigment is not removed.

SOLUTIONS:

- Buffer formalin solutions to a pH of 6.8 to 7.4.
- Treat tissues with iodine and sodium thiosulfate to remove mercury pigment.

COMMENTS: It is almost impossible to totally prevent formalin pigment from forming in very bloody tissues or in sections that have been decalcified and not washed well in running water; however, the use of buffered formalin solutions will go a long way in preventing this pigment from forming. Formalin pigment has the ability to reduce silver solution and therefore will stain with some silver techniques. It can be removed, when necessary, by treating the sections with an alcoholic solution of picric acid. Mercury pigment is easily removed with iodine and sodium thiosulfate and should not be present in the stained sections.

PROBLEM: Nuclear Bubbling

APPEARANCE: Nuclei look as if they contain soap-suds; the chromatin pattern is disturbed and bubbly (Figures 1.19 and 1.20).

CAUSE:

- Incomplete fixation with formalin.

SOLUTION:

- Ensure that the specimen is fixed adequately before processing.

COMMENTS: Although this artifact has traditionally been thought of as a fixation artifact, it also can occur when sections are picked up from the flotation bath and not drained well before they are dried in a hot dryer or in the microwave oven.

Decalcification

Decalcification is a procedure used daily in the majority of histopathology laboratories and frequently yields suboptimal results. Often, the time allowed for specimen fixation, the choice of decalcification reagent, and the time allowed for decalcification are not the best; it also may be a combination of these factors. Unless the decalcification reagent is combined with a fixative, the specimen must be fixed prior to decalcification. Many decalcification reagents are available, and each should be used differently according to the type or chemical formulation. However, it is the time allowed for the decalcification process that is the most important factor for achieving excellent preparations, as underdecalcified tissue will be difficult to cut, and overdecalcified tissue will most likely show a loss of basophilic staining properties. Some decalcification reagents, like hydrochloric and nitric acid solutions, are very strong and act very rapidly, while others, like formic acid and EDTA solutions, are

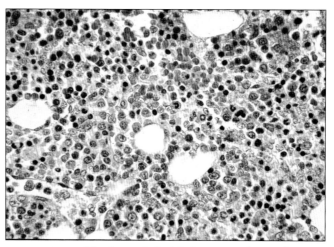

Figure 1.21. A well-fixed, properly decalcified specimen is shown in this image, with excellent preservation of nuclear detail and good cytoplasmic differentiation. (From Carson FL. *Histotechnology: A Self-Instructional Text.* 2nd ed. © 1997 American Society of Clinical Pathologists. Reproduced with permission.)

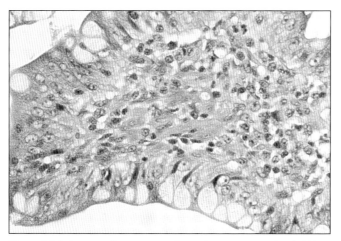

Figure 1.19. A section of gastrointestinal tract demonstrating nuclear bubbling, most often a result of inadequate formalin fixation.[3]

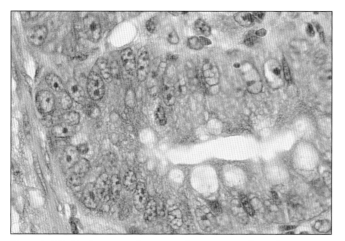

Figure 1.20. A higher power of a section of gastrointestinal tract demonstrating nuclear bubbling; there is a soap-suds appearance in the nuclei.[3]

milder formulations and act slowly, so the end point of exposure to these reagents must be carefully and frequently monitored. In many laboratories, the end point is determined by simply flexing the tissue, which is not optimal or accurate, and may generate internal artifacts. The presence of calcium ions in the decalcification solution can be determined by adding a solution containing ammonium hydroxide and ammonium oxalate. This method requires that each specimen be placed in a separate container and that the solution be changed after each end point check. Using a radiographic unit is the most exact method of determining the end point of decalcification, and since there are small radiographic units available in many histology laboratories, it is the method of choice, especially for specimens on which the end point is in doubt. The final important step in the decalcification process requires that the tissue be thoroughly washed to neutralize and remove excess acid.

A well-fixed, properly decalcified specimen will show excellent preservation of the nuclear detail, a lack of calcium in the bony spicules, and good cytoplasmic differentiation, as demonstrated in Figure 1.21. Although no bony spicules are shown in this figure, the nuclear detail is excellent, with the more open chromatin patterns of the white cell precursors and the dense chromatin patterns of the red cell precursors well demonstrated. Some cytoplasmic differentiation is also apparent. There is moderate lysis of the mature red blood cells due to the presence of acetic acid in the fixative.

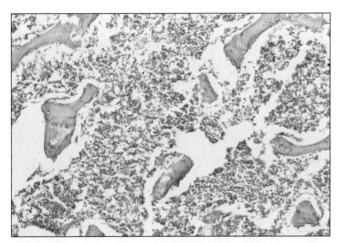

Figure 1.22. A section of bone demonstrating overdecalcification; all nuclear detail is lost.

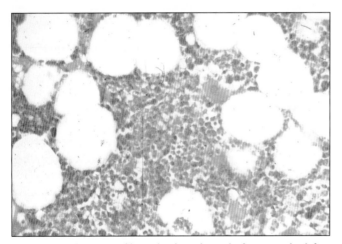

Figure 1.23. This section of bone also shows the result of excessive decalcification; differential nuclear and cytoplasmic staining is absent.

Problems Encountered With Decalcification

PROBLEM: Excessive Decalcification

APPEARANCE: Excessive decalcification results in a loss of nuclear detail, a decrease in basophilic staining properties, and finally a complete loss of nuclear staining (Figures 1.22 and 1.23).

CAUSES:

- Sections left in decalcification solution for too long a period of time.
- Sections not well fixed before placing in decalcification solution.

SOLUTIONS:

- Rigorously monitor the end point of decalcification, using radiography if necessary.
- Ensure good fixation before placing sections in decalcification solution, or use a decalcification solution that contains a fixative.

PROBLEM: Inadequate Decalcification

APPEARANCE: Areas of the tissue section containing unremoved calcium will stain dark blue with hematoxylin (Figure 1.24).

CAUSES:

- Section was not placed in decalcifying fluid before processing.
- Section was left in decalcifying solution for too little time.

SOLUTIONS:

- Ensure that tissues containing calcium are placed in decalcifying fluid. If areas of residual calcification are noted when sectioning a block, surface decalcification can be done by carefully facing the block, and then treating the exposed face with a decalcifying fluid for 30 to 60 minutes. The block must then be rinsed well, and the first ribbon taken.
- Check the end point of decalcification carefully; use radiography if necessary to determine completeness of decalcification.

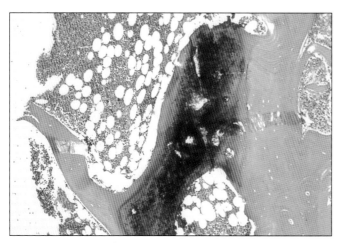

Figure 1.24. A section of bone that has not been completely decalcified.

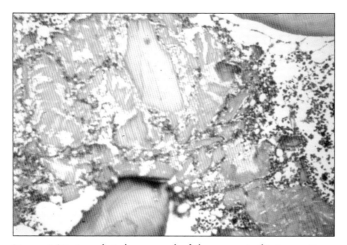

Figure 1.25. Bone dust obscures much of the marrow in this image. (From: Carson FL. *Histotechnology: A Self-Instructional Text.* 2nd ed. © 1997 American Society of Clinical Pathologists. Reproduced with permission.)

PROBLEM: Bone Dust

APPEARANCE: Bony debris obscures parts of the section (Figure 1.25).

CAUSE:

- Bone debris is pressed into the surface of the bone by the saw.

SOLUTIONS:

- Use a saw with a diamond blade to obtain the section.
- Cut the original specimen thick, and then trim the surfaces following decalcification.

Embedding

There are two especially important factors that are to be considered when embedding tissues. The first is specimen orientation. Several methods have been proposed to aid in this critical process, for example, ink dotting or notching the top of the specimen. These methods work on large specimens but are ineffective on smaller specimens. With the widespread use of inks to mark margins, ink dotting to indicate the top of the specimen is no longer popular. When larger tissues have been properly fixed and grossed, there is rarely an orientation problem. Many laboratories use a grossing list or worksheet, which may be used as a reference while embedding. It is also helpful to note any special embedding instructions, such as "tube," "edge," or "skin," on the side of the cassette. Another practice involves using an Embedding Alert form to call attention to particularly fragile or problematic specimens with complex embedding instructions. Such a form would accompany the work list and/or processed specimen(s) to the embedding station for easy reference by the histologist.

The second problem, which occurs with large specimens or with multiple fragments, is embedding all of the tissue(s) at the same level so that sectioning will reveal a good cross-section of everything in the block. Pressing down the single specimen until it adheres to the bottom of the mold, or keeping the paraffin melted until multiple pieces can be transferred to the mold and then pressing on each piece as the paraffin cools, will usually achieve even, flat embedding. This is especially critical when dealing with tiny-gauge needle biopsies. With multiple pieces of small tissues, it is easy to miss a piece and leave it in the cassette or to find it stuck to the cassette lid. The histologist should make a consistent practice of carefully checking each lid for tissue at the time the lid is removed and before it is discarded. In a similar potential problem situation, the histologist must exercise great care when opening bagged or wrapped tiny specimens in order to prevent them from "launching" onto the table, floor, or a lab coat. Whenever working with multiple tissue pieces, it is helpful to write the number of pieces on the side of the cassette so that they may be counted during embedding. Good embedding technique comes with practice.

One final excellent embedding practice requires that the forceps be thoroughly cleaned and inspected for tissue residue between specimens. This action will prevent critical errors related to tissue transfer from one case to another and the possibility of an incorrect diagnosis.

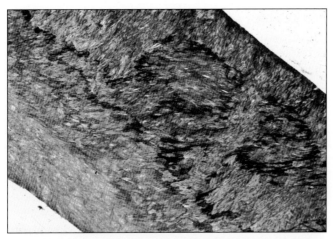

Figure 1.26. A Verhoeff-Van Gieson–stained section of aorta has been embedded flat rather than on edge, so that the usual parallel elastic lamina are not seen.

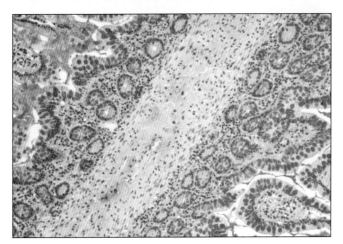

Figure 1.27. This Alcian blue–stained section of intestine was most likely not well fixed before grossing, so that it has rolled and all layers cannot be seen.

Problems Encountered With Embedding

PROBLEM: Poor Section Orientation

APPEARANCE: All layers are not demonstrated on tissues that have walls or layers, such as gastrointestinal specimens or skin. The lumen cannot be seen on tubular structures, such as fallopian tube or arteries (Figures 1.26 and 1.27).

CAUSES:
- Poor specimen embedding technique.
- Tissue incompletely fixed and hardened before grossing, so that the layers have rolled.

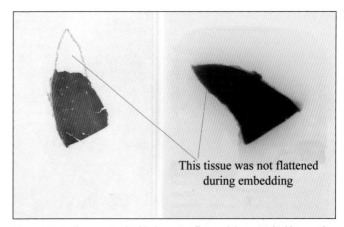

This tissue was not flattened during embedding

Figure 1.28. The tissue in this block was not flattened during embedding, so that a complete section has not been obtained. Deeper cutting may result in a complete section, but there is also a risk of cutting through a part of the tissue that was embedded at a deeper level.

SOLUTIONS:
- Become familiar with tissue identification by observing grossing process.
- Always refer to embedding instructions on the cassette or grossing worksheet.
- Orient tissue carefully when embedding, noting tissue type.
- Ensure that tissue adheres evenly to the bottom of the embedding mold.
- Ensure that tissue is hardened enough by fixation so that it does not roll during grossing.

PROBLEM: A Complete Cross-Section Is Not Obtained on All Tissue in the Block

APPEARANCE: When matched to the block, the slide shows that only part of the tissue has been sectioned (Figure 1.28).

CAUSES:
- The tissue section has not been pressed flat in the embedding mold.
- The paraffin has been allowed to chill as multiple fragments are embedded.

SOLUTIONS:
- Ensure that the tissue is pressed flat in the mold during embedding.
- Do not allow the paraffin to cool until all fragments are in the mold, then press on each as the paraffin chills.
- Use embedding tools such as spatulas, tampers, or stampers to ensure proper embedding depth and flattening.

References

1. Carson FL. *Histotechnology: A Self-Instructional Text.* 2nd ed. Chicago, IL: American Society of Clinical Pathologists; 1997:90-95.

2. Feldman A. *H&E Stain. NSH-CAP HQIP. A Final Critique.* Northfield IL: College of American Pathologists; 2004: 20-26.

3. Dapson RW. *Spotlight on practice: fixation. NSH-CAP HQIP. A Final Critique.* Northfield IL: College of American Pathologists; 2004: 14-19.

4. Wynnchuk M. Evaluation of xylene substitutes for paraffin tissue processing. *J Histotechnol.* 1994;17:143.

5. Wright KR. Research antigen retrieval solution. *J Histotechnol.* 1994;17:81.

ACKNOWLEDGEMENT:
Thank you to Dr. Richard Dapson, who wrote the original fixation paper for a NSH/CAP HistoQIP Final Critique (see reference). The majority of the introductory material on fixation for this chapter is taken directly from that paper, as are several of the images.

Microtomy

Freida L. Carson
Robert L. Lott

One of the critical steps in the production of high-quality microscopic sections is microtomy. It is primarily an acquired manual skill that demands experience. Although the experience and training of the microtomist is very important, good sections cannot be produced without excellent equipment. One needs a microtome that is well adjusted, clean, and free of vibration in any of its parts; a very sharp blade that is free of defect along the edge and properly installed at the correct angle; and some means of chilling the paraffin blocks. Worn or poorly maintained microtome parts can cause thick and thin sections or microscopic chatter, especially in very dense tissues. Most routine sections are cut at a micrometer setting of approximately 4 μm. Although there is a micrometer setting on the microtome, it is not absolute. How thick the sections really are depends on many factors, such as the nature of the paraffin used for embedding and the temperature of the paraffin block being sectioned. Regardless of how sharp the blade is, a correct clearance angle, or the angle between the cutting facet of the knife and the block face, is critical. If this angle, usually between 5 and 10 degrees, is not properly set, it can result in thick sections, skipped sections, compression, and microscopic chatter. Before paraffin blocks are sectioned, they should be chilled. The purpose of chilling is to harden the paraffin polymers and aid in cutting dense, hard, or very fibrous tissues. Soft tissues, on the other hand, are often cut more easily and without wrinkling if the block is not too cold. Some histologists prefer to face the blocks and then chill them for sectioning. After facing a block, it is placed face down on ice or in ice water for additional cooling time, and then the block is microfaced to smooth any rough edges before beginning to "ribbon."

As sections are cut, ideally the leading edge of one section will adhere to the latter edge of the previous section, forming a ribbon. This ribbon is then detached from the knife and floated on a water bath, where it is stretched slightly to rid the section of folds, wrinkles, and compression. The temperature of this water bath is usually about 10° to 12°F below the melting point of the paraffin used. An overheated water bath or excessive stretching of the sections will produce artifactual separation of tissue components, mimicking edema. The sec-

tion is then picked up on a glass slide, allowed to drain briefly, and dried. Draining of the slides before drying is important, because if too much water is on or under the section when the slide is placed in a hot dryer, an artifact known as "nuclear bubbling" may result. Sections may be air-dried overnight, dried in an oven, or dried in a forced-air drier designed for that purpose. Although some laboratories dry sections using a microwave, this method is not recommended.

There must be some method of ensuring that the section will stay on the slide during the staining process. Adhesives may be added to the water bath, or slides may be coated with, or dipped in, some type of adhesive. Recently, positively charged slides have become available, and many laboratories are employing these slides in techniques that are notorious for causing the loss of sections.

Defects in sections caused by poor or improper microtomy techniques can present diagnostic problems for the pathologist reading the section. The majority of these problems can be prevented during microtomy with awareness and care on the part of the microtomist. Over the first six of the NSH/CAP HistoQIP (HQIP) challenges, an external quality assurance program developed by the National Society for Histotechnology and the College of American Pathologists, the hematoxylin-and-eosin (H&E)–stained sections from an average of 57% of laboratories contained artifacts that kept them from achieving the best score possible. These percentages varied from a low of 44% on lung sections to a high of 76% on lymph node sections.

Table 2.1 shows the five most common microtomy artifacts in the first eight H&E challenges of the HQIP program. The percentages are based on the total number of H&E slides submitted for each tissue type. These artifacts, along with some of the other more common microtomy defects, are described and illustrated along with corrective or preventive measures. The images were chosen to best demonstrate the artifact and may or may not represent good staining.

No section demonstrating what should be seen in a well-cut section is presented because it is obvious that a section demonstrating good microtomy technique will be artifact free.

Table 2.1. The Most Common Microtomy Artifacts in the First Eight HQIP H&E Challenges

Tissue H&E	% Wrinkles/ Folds	% Tears/ Fragmented	% Holes	% Knife Lines	% Thick
Breast	19	8	11	3	5
Skin	24	12	10	5	3
Lymph Node	30	29	22	17	20
Lung	20	10	5	3	9
Uterus	30	13	17	9	7
Colon	43	23	20	17	5
Bone Marrow	28	18	7	2	15
Liver	43	23	20	17	5
Average	**30**	**17**	**14**	**9**	**9**

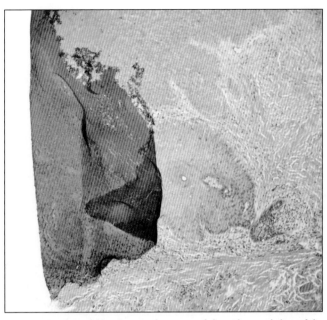

Figure 2.2. A large fold is shown in this section of skin. The morphology of the tissue is obscured by this type of artifact.

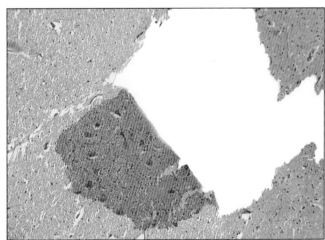

Figure 2.3. One portion of this section of brain tissue has detached from the slide and then folded over, masking the morphology in that area.

Problems Encountered With Microtomy

PROBLEM: Wrinkles/Folds

APPEARANCE: Although both of these artifacts are commonly referred to as folds, wrinkles involve three layers of tissue overlying one another, whereas folds involve only two layers of tissue. Wrinkles represent an accordion-like layering of the section and tend to occur within the central areas of the tissue (Figure 2.1), where-

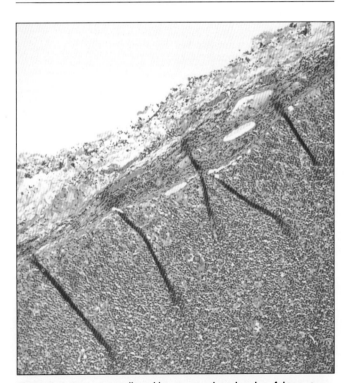

Figure 2.1. Numerous small wrinkles are seen along the edge of this section.

as folds usually occur when one edge of the tissue is folded over onto the remainder of the section (Figures 2.2 and 2.3).

CAUSES:

- Not stretching the tissue sufficiently on the water bath.
- Improper temperature of the water bath.
- Tissue not adhered well to the slide.

SOLUTIONS:

- Gently stretch the tissue and tease out wrinkles and folds while the tissue section is on the water bath.
- Check the temperature of the water bath. Sections will not spread appropriately when too cold; if too hot, wrinkles or folds may result as soon as the tissue touches the water.
- Adjust the temperature to optimize softening of paraffin within the section to promote tissue stretching.
- Ensure that the tissue will adhere to the slide by using adhesives or positively charged slides.

PROBLEM: Tears/Fragmentation

APPEARANCE: There is disruption in the tissue morphology, or a torn or fragmented section occurs.

CAUSES:

- Incompletely fixed and processed tissue, causing disintegration on the water bath (Figure 2.4).
- Overstretching on the water bath (Figure 2.5).
- Temperature of the water bath is too high.
- Tearing with instruments used during sectioning or coverslipping (Figure 2.6).

SOLUTIONS:

- Ensure complete fixation and processing.
- Gently stretch ribbons on the water bath to remove wrinkles and folds.
- Decrease temperature of the water bath.
- Carefully handle ribbons with metal instruments during sectioning and flotation.
- Keep other slides or instruments from touching sections after they are mounted on slides.

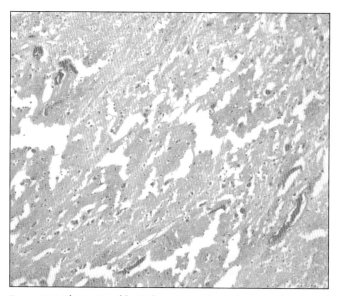

Figure 2.4. This section of brain demonstrates the result of poor fixation and processing; it has disintegrated on the water bath.

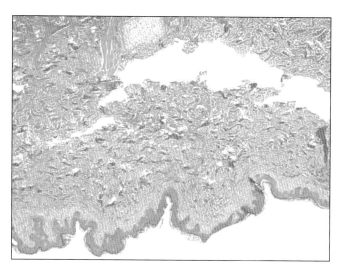

Figure 2.5. A large tear is seen in this section of skin, most likely caused by overstretching on the water bath.

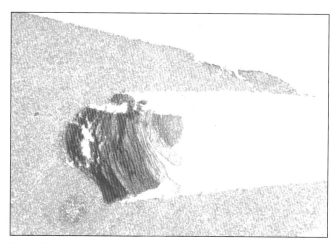

Figure 2.6. The result of tearing with instruments can be seen in this section.

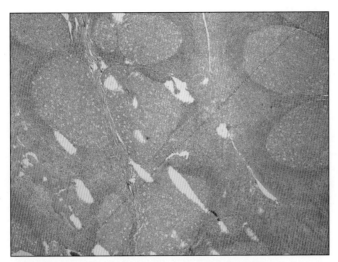

Figure 2.7. Multiple holes can be seen in this section of tonsil.

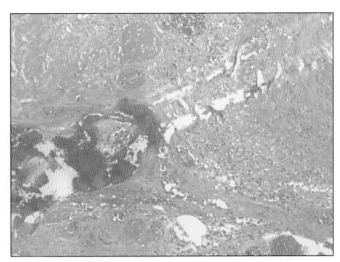

Figure 2.9. A large area of calcification has caused a knife line that is carried through the remainder of the section.

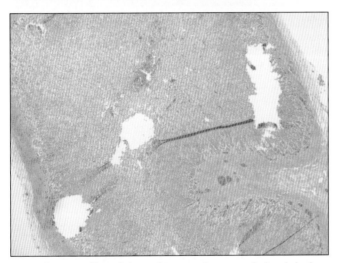

Figure 2.8. Several large holes can be seen in this section of adrenal gland.

PROBLEM: Holes

APPEARANCE: There are irregularly shaped holes ("moth-eaten effect") that disappear as the block is ribboned (Figures 2.7 and 2.8).

CAUSE:

- This problem can result from aggressive trimming of the block during sectioning. The holes are caused by the actual removal of small pieces of tissue, which can occur with any tissue block, but is particularly common in liver, tonsil, lymph node, spleen, and brain. Rarely, holes may be caused by a dull knife.

SOLUTIONS:

- Gently and carefully face the tissue block, decrease micrometer setting, add moisture to the block face via moist gauze or cotton ball, place block back on the ice bath or moisten thumb and apply to the surface of the block, and then make a continuous ribbon using smooth, even strokes until the artifact disappears (this technique is dependent upon the quantity of tissue in the block).
- Ensure that the knife is sharp.

PROBLEM: Knife Lines / Scratches

APPEARANCE: Knife lines or scratches appear as vertical lines or tissue disruptions usually running completely through each section.

CAUSES:

- Hard particles in tissue (calcified areas or crystals) or foreign material, such as staples or sutures (Figures 2.9 and 2.10).
- Nicks in the knife.
- Lint or paraffin lying on the edge of the knife (Figure 2.11).
- Impurities in the paraffin.

SOLUTIONS:

- Change the knife or move to a new area of the blade.
- Use surface decalcification methods.
- Carefully clean edge of knife to remove excess paraffin buildup.
- If there is foreign material in the paraffin, re-embed with clean paraffin.

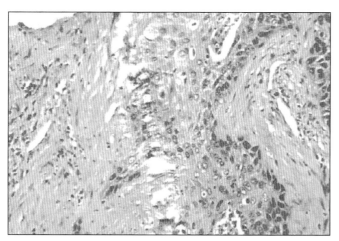

Figure 2.10. A jagged knife line can be seen in this section, possibly caused by a foreign body, such as a suture, in the tissue.

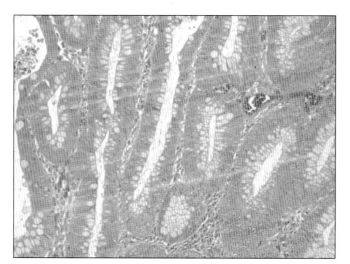

Figure 2.11. Paraffin on the knife edge is one cause of the knife lines seen in this section; another is small flaws produced in the knife edge by cleaning. The tissue is not disrupted, but simply scored.

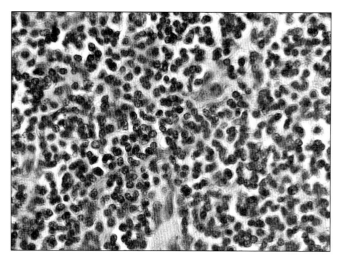

Figure 2.12. This section is very thick, with more than two layers of nuclei apparent.

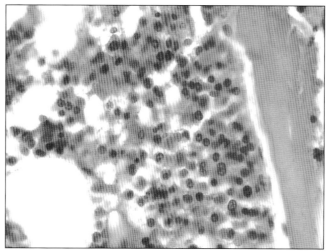

Figure 2.13. This section of bone marrow demonstrates more than one layer of nuclei.

PROBLEM: Section Is Too Thick

APPEARANCE: Two definite layers of cell nuclei can be seen when focusing up and down (Figures 2.12 and 2.13).

CAUSES:
- Improperly maintained microtome.
- Wrong micrometer setting.
- Paraffin too soft (melting point too low).
- Paraffin too warm.
- Dull knife.

SOLUTIONS:
- Decrease micrometer setting.
- Maintain microtomes according to manufacturer's recommendations, including periodic calibration and lubrication.
- Use paraffin with melting point that is appropriate to tissue type and density.

COMMENTS: The clinical standard for routine tissue sections is 3 to 5 μm thick, with 3 to 4 μm being preferred. Exceptions to this include kidney biopsies, which are usually cut at 2 μm; central nervous system tissues, which are usually cut at 8 μm; and tissues for some special stains. Properly serviced, clean, and well-maintained equipment is vital to producing sections that conform to the micrometer setting of the instrument. Cooling of paraffin blocks is also important in good microtomy, because contact between the block face and knife generates friction (heat) and can cause expansion of the block. A section cut at a setting of 5 μm can actually be 6 to 7 μm thick under the influence of this friction.

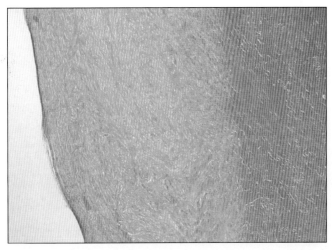

Figure 2.14. The staining in this image appears uneven, caused by a thick-and-thin section.

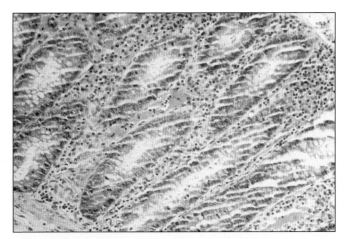

Figure 2.15. This section of gastrointestinal tract demonstrates the microscopic chatter most often caused by cutting too rapidly. With most tissues, better sections are obtained when the knife passes the block face about once each second.

PROBLEM: Variable or Thick-and-Thin Sections

APPEARANCE: Part of the section is thick and part is thin (Figure 2.14), showing a characteristic light-and-dark staining with an irregular pattern; or one section is thick and the next is thin.

CAUSES:

- Too little knife tilt or clearance angle too small.
- Worn microtome parts.
- Incorrectly maintained microtomes that are not regularly oiled and calibrated.
- Cutting very dense tissue.
- Loose block or knife, or knife tightened down too much; paraffin remaining on block edges, preventing adequate tightening of the block holder.

SOLUTIONS:

- Check all microtome screws/clamps to ensure that the knife is correctly tightened.
- Check that the block is firmly held.
- Increase knife angle.
- Maintain microtomes according to manufacturer's recommendations, including periodic calibration and lubrication.
- Remove excess paraffin from edges of blocks.

PROBLEM: Chatter/"Venetian Blind"/Washboarding

APPEARANCE: Parallel thick and thin areas occur in the section, or there is separation of the tissue section into fine lines. These artifacts often occur in small gastrointestinal biopsies, cervical biopsies, and other glandular tissues (Figures 2.15 and 2.16).

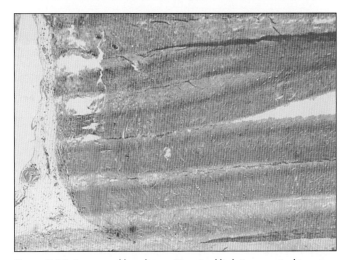

Figure 2.16. Severe washboarding or "Venetian blinds," as seen in this section, is most often caused by a worn or loose microtome part, or by an improperly clamped block.

CAUSES:

- Overdehydration of the tissue during processing.
- Dull knife.
- Too much knife tilt, or clearance angle too great.
- Cutting too rapidly.
- Loose or worn microtome parts, including loose block or knife holder.
- Dense or compact tissue.

SOLUTIONS:

- Use less dehydration time during processing.
- Soak block face with wet cotton or by dipping thumb in water bath and rubbing the block face.
- Decrease knife tilt.
- Decrease cutting speed.
- Ensure that the knife and block are tightened securely.

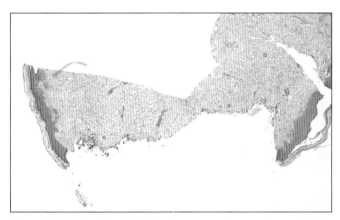

Figure 2.17. This section of skin has been cut too deep, so that much of the epidermis and dermis have been cut away. This extremely serious error is not correctable.

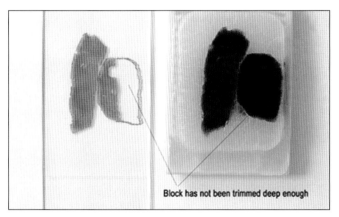

Figure 2.18. A representative section of the tissue in the block has not been obtained by the microtomist, which is an error that could have serious consequences.

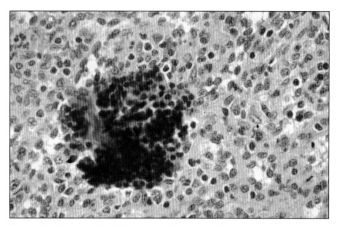

Figure 2.19. Tissue debris has been picked up on this section.

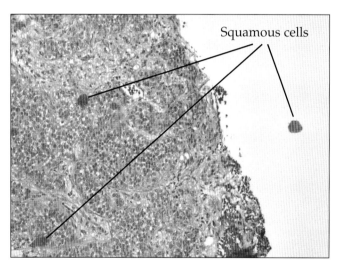

Figure 2.20. Several squamous cells can be seen lying on the tissue or slide in this section.

PROBLEM: Incomplete Tissue Section

APPEARANCE: This artifact is most obvious in sections with an epithelial surface (ie, skin) when the epithelium is incomplete; it is often picked up when stained sections are matched to the block face (Figures 2.17 and 2.18).

CAUSES:

- Incorrect embedding so that the tissue is not flat in the block.
- Not cutting deep enough into the block.
- Cutting too deep into the block.

SOLUTIONS:

- Ensure that the tissue is evenly flattened in the embedding mold.
- Face the block so that a complete section of the tissue is exposed before beginning to ribbon.
- Ensure that a section is taken before cutting too deep into the block.
- Match stained sections with blocks to ensure that a complete section was obtained.

PROBLEM: Floaters/Debris

APPEARANCE: Material, such as squamous epithelial cells or other cellular debris, is deposited on top of the tissue section or on the slide underneath the section (Figures 2.19 and 2.20).

CAUSES:

- Debris in the water bath, such as squamous cells from dandruff or from dry skin of the hands.
- Cellular material from previous sections left on the water bath.

SOLUTIONS:

- Clean the water bath by skimming paper towels (or similar material) across the surface of the bath between blocks.
- If poorly fixed tissue has "exploded" on the bath, change the solution in the bath before sectioning other cases; this may also be necessary after sectioning bloody tissues.

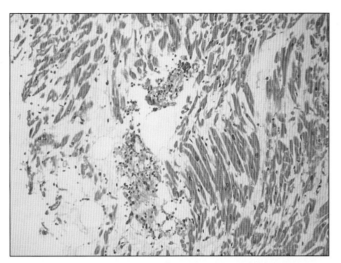

Figure 2.21. A contaminant from another tissue source can be seen in the upper middle of this section of cardiac muscle.

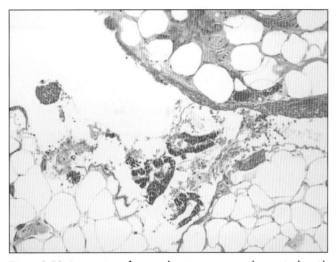

Figure 2.22. A contaminant from another tissue source can be seen in the middle of this section of adipose tissue.

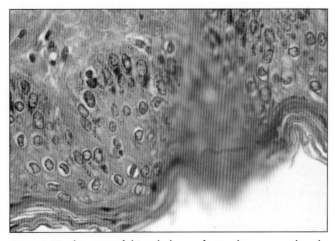

Figure 2.23. This section of skin at high magnification shows a wave along the edge, making it impossible to focus on the section all in one plane.

PROBLEM: Contamination From Other Tissue Sources ("Floaters")—An Extremely Serious Problem

APPEARANCE: Tissue from one patient may contaminate sections from a different patient and may be impossible to recognize if of the same tissue type. Contaminants are often from tissues known to be highly friable when sectioned, such as chorionic villi, large colon polyps, and testicular tumors (Figures 2.21 and 2.22).

CAUSES:
- Improperly maintained and cleaned water bath.
- Tissue carryover at either the grossing table or the embedding station.
- Failure to wrap friable tissues before placing in the cassette.

SOLUTIONS:
- Meticulously clean instruments used for grossing—especially forceps—between each case.
- Between blocks, meticulously clean instruments used for embedding.
- Wrap friable tissues in tea bags or equivalent before processing.
- Clean water bath between cases/blocks; if improperly fixed and/or processed tissue explodes on the water bath, clean bath and change flotation solution.

COMMENTS: This situation is a very serious error that often originates before microtomy begins. Instruments used for grossing one specimen can carry over contaminants to another, or forceps used for embedding one specimen may contaminate another. It can also happen during microtomy. Awareness is the key, along with good habits of cleaning instruments between specimens and keeping the water bath scrupulously clean. Poorly processed tissues that explode on the bath can leave debris behind that is sometimes difficult to remove by skimming the bath surface. In this case, the water must be changed.

PROBLEM: Wavy Section

APPEARANCE: The section is not in focus all in one plane. This artifact frequently occurs with skin sections (Figure 2.23).

CAUSES:
- Incomplete flattening on the water bath.
- Improper water bath temperature.
- "Overprocessed" tissue that is hard and brittle to cut, which often leads to poor adhesion to the slide.

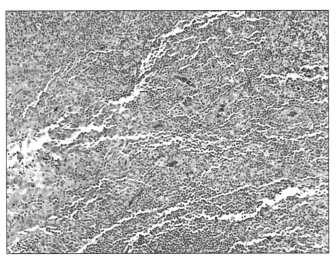

Figure 2.24. Numerous cracks are present in this section, most likely resulting from poor fixation. This artifact is also known as "parched earth" because of its resemblance to extremely dry soil.

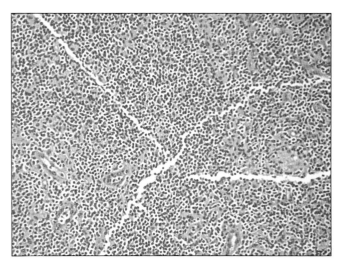

Figure 2.25. Numerous cracks are present in this section, most likely resulting from suboptimal fixation and processing.

SOLUTIONS:

- Allow for longer time on the water bath.
- Try for better stretching of the ribbon as it is put on the bath.
- Check temperature of water bath.

PROBLEM: Cracks/"Parched-Earth" Appearance

APPEARANCE: There are irregular cracks in the tissue, resembling those that occur in the earth during periods of drought.

CAUSES:

- Incomplete fixation (Figure 2.24).
- Inadequate clearing and paraffin infiltration.
- High temperature of the water bath.
- Excessive dehydration, which can remove protein-bound water, creating tissue that is brittle and may crack when floated out (Figure 2.25).
- Overuse of coolant spray during sectioning (Figure 2.26).

SOLUTIONS:

- Ensure adequate fixation, dehydration, clearing, and infiltration.
- Lower the temperature of the water bath.
- Do not use coolant spray during sectioning.

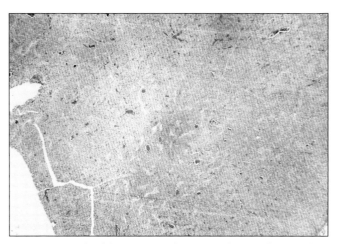

Figure 2.26. Cracks of the type seen in this poor reticulin stain often result from using cryosprays, which can fracture the surface of the paraffin block.

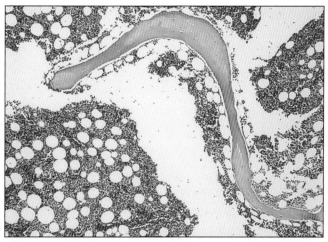

Figure 2.27. Extreme separation of the marrow elements can be seen in this section of bone marrow.

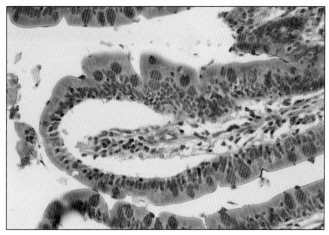

Figure 2.28. The lamina propria has completely retracted from the epithelium in this section of small intestine.

PROBLEM: Extreme Separation of Tissue Elements

APPEARANCE: Tissue elements are separated by wide, clear spaces (Figures 2.27 and 2.28).

CAUSES:

- Overstretching of tissue on the water bath.
- Floating tissues for too long.
- Not allowing cut sections to drain well before placing in dryer.

SOLUTION:

- Stretch and/or float tissue only enough to flatten and get rid of wrinkles; do not overstretch or prolong flotation.
- Allow cut sections to drain well before drying.

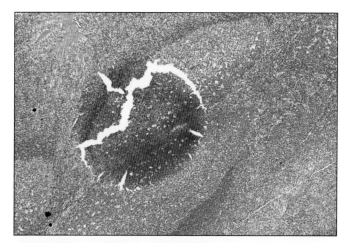

Figure 2.29. An air bubble was trapped under this section when it was picked up from the water bath. The bubble broke during drying or staining, and that area accepted stain on top of and underneath the section, causing the area of the bubble to exhibit a more intense stain.

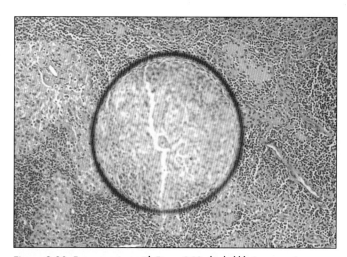

Figure 2.30. For comparison with Figure 2.29, this bubble is a mounting or coverslipping artifact. Air was trapped under the coverslip during mounting, and the area of the bubble is lighter and out of focus.

PROBLEM: Bubbles

APPEARANCE: Bubbles occurring during microtomy appear as circular areas in the section that are stained more intensely than the surrounding area (Figure 2.29); this is in contrast to an air bubble trapped under the coverslip during mounting (Figure 2.30), which stains less intensely.

CAUSE:

- Air bubbles are trapped under the section when it is picked up from the water bath. The bubble breaks during drying or staining, and that area tends to accept stain both on top of and underneath the section, causing the area of the bubble to exhibit a more intense stain.

SOLUTIONS:

- Fill a large flask with the water for the water bath and allow it to stand overnight before pouring it into the bath, allowing all air to escape.
- Stir the water in the bath if bubbles seem to be forming on the bottom.

Bibliography

Carson FL. *Histotechnology: A Self-Instructional Text.* 2nd ed. Chicago, IL: American Society of Clinical Pathologists; 1997.

Sheehan DC, Hrapchak BB. *Theory and Practice of Histotechnology.* 2nd ed. Columbus, OH: Battelle Press; 1980.

Frozen Sections

Vinnie Della Speranza

The preparation of sections from frozen unfixed tissue has important applications in clinical and research environments. Some tissue constituents can only be studied in frozen sections, as they are removed or denatured during routine tissue processing. These include lipids and a variety of labile enzymes. Other constituents, such as glycogen, may be artifactually displaced from their sites of origin during fixation or processing, making their study advantageous in frozen sections. Immunofluorescence techniques are likewise carried out on frozen sections. Such studies aside, the clinical laboratory relies heavily on the frozen section technique to provide intraoperative consultations when the surgeon requires a rapid diagnosis or immediate feedback relating to surgical margins. As a result, virtually all clinical and many research laboratories utilize frozen section cryotomy to support their work.

Many of the principles of routine paraffin microtomy apply to frozen-section cryotomy; these have been discussed at length in chapter 2. Attention to details such as microtome blade bevel angle and block face clearance angle apply equally to any microtomy procedure. However, most would agree that the unique characteristics of frozen tissue pose a greater challenge for histology personnel involved in the preparation of frozen sections. Successful sectioning of frozen tissues requires:
- Properly embedded and frozen samples
- A well-maintained instrument in good operating order
- A clean, sharp, microtome blade that is firmly secured in the instrument blade holder and set at the proper clearance angle
- A temperature appropriate for the tissue being sectioned
- A specimen firmly attached to a specimen chuck that is firmly clamped in the microtome
- A skilled technologist

Section quality is largely dependent upon tissue freezing technique and the skill of the cryotome operator. Section quality rivaling that commonly attained with routine paraffin sections is highly achievable if one is prepared to invest the time needed to become expert in this technique. This will require knowledge of cryotome operation, including the use of anti-roll devices, proper embedding and freezing technique, and the optimal cutting temperatures for various tissue types.

Where optimal tissue preservation and cellular morphology are required, snap freezing of tissues at ultra-low temperatures (approximately -80°C or lower) is necessary. A number of techniques have been described in the literature, but the most prevalent include the use of liquid-nitrogen–chilled isopentane (2-methylbutane) or isopentane chilled in dry ice. In these methods, a beaker of isopentane is immersed in liquid nitrogen (or dry ice) until the isopentane begins to freeze; the appearance of white ice in the bottom of the beaker indicates that the isopentane has reached a temperature of approximately -150°C. At this time, a mold containing cryomedium-embedded tissue can be lowered into the isopentane to effect freezing (see Figure 3.1). As an alternative, one may prepare a dry ice/solvent (acetone or isopentane) slurry in which tissues to be frozen are immersed. An excellent review by Callis[1] discusses a variety of freezing techniques in greater detail. In addition, commercially available electrical units capable of rapidly freezing blocks in super-chilled isopentane or similar organic solvents are now used in many clinical laboratories.

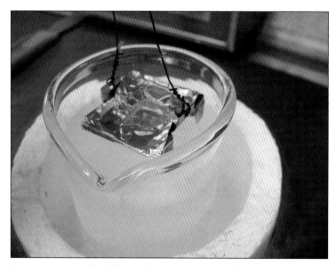

Figure 3.1. A metal mold lined with aluminum foil will efficiently conduct the low temperature of the isopentane. The mold is filled with cryoembedding medium, and the sample is pressed to the bottom of the mold, which will become the cutting surface of the block.

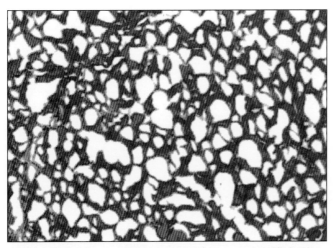

Figure 3.2. Slow freezing techniques can result in a sample riddled with ice crystals (ice crystal or freezing artifact). This section of skeletal muscle is virtually unrecognizable.

Due to the very rapid freezing these techniques allow, one is able to avoid the introduction of ice crystal (freezing) artifact, which is commonly seen when slower freezing techniques are utilized. Ice crystal artifact is the appearance of discontinuous tissue architecture resulting from component displacement when interstitial water freezes in situ. As the water freezes, it expands and displaces surrounding tissues. At times this artifact can be so severe as to cause the appearance of multiple gaps or holes in the tissue, rendering the sample unsuitable for morphologic study (Figure 3.2).

Some laboratories choose to freeze their tissues directly inside the cryostat on the freezing platform or "cryobar," which is maintained near -30° to -50°C in most instruments (Figures 3.3 and 3.4). By placing the specimen chuck onto the cryobar and using a heat extractor on the block face, one can achieve freezing simultaneously from both the block face and the block holder; this technique freezes the sample quickly and thoroughly. This technique will not provide the quality typically required in the research laboratory, but it is adequate for the clinical laboratory needing to provide rapid consultation to the operating room.

Tissue is often frozen in the cryostat in the interest of time as the sample will end up at sectioning temperature, while tissues snap frozen in chilled isopentane are too cold for immediate sectioning and must be "warmed" to cryostat temperature before sectioning can be undertaken.[2] While cryostat-frozen samples are more prone to freezing artifact, this can be reduced by keeping the cryoembedding medium cold in a refrigerator and keeping the specimen chucks cold (these may be stored in the cryostat on the cryobar). Both of these strategies will speed up block freezing in the cryostat and will reduce the amount of artifact. Some tissues, such as brain, lung, kidney, and bowel, may be especially prone

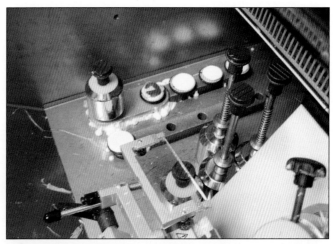

Figure 3.3. Tissue to be frozen is placed onto a cold cryostat chuck previously coated with cryoembedding medium. After placement of the tissue, the chuck is returned to the cryostat to complete freezing. Skill and practice are required in order to achieve a flat block face with the entire sample in a single plane. In inexperienced hands, tissues may be frozen in different planes within the block, setting the stage for tissue to be lost during trimming in an attempt to achieve a full face section representative of the entire sample.

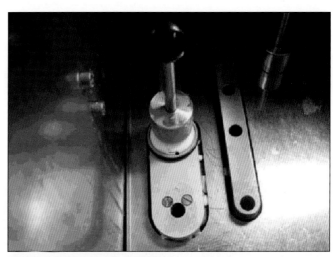

Figure 3.4. A heat extractor is applied on top of the tissue in order to speed up freezing and achieve a flat block face.

to artifact; if time allows, this can be reduced by pre-chilling the specimen in a refrigerator prior to embedding and freezing.[3]

A number of cryoembedding media are available commercially. It is important to recognize that the properties of these media may well be different at cryotome temperatures, since most cryoembedding formulations are proprietary. Some cryoembedding media section more easily at colder temperatures (-25°C or colder), while others may become brittle at colder temperatures. Therefore, each laboratory should evaluate available products to determine their sectioning characteristics and their suitability for the intended applications.

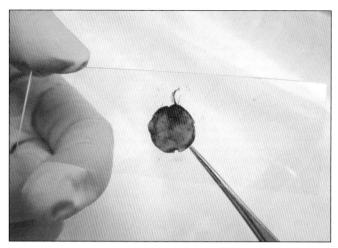

Figure 3.5. A glass slide may be used as a freezing platform to achieve proper specimen orientation and a flat block face. The tissue is laid out and oriented with the understanding that the side adherent to the glass will become the surface that is sectioned.

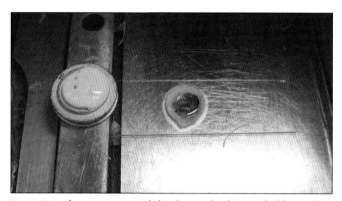

Figure 3.6. The tissue is surrounded and covered with cryoembedding medium to prevent drying, and the slide is placed onto a cold metal surface inside the cryostat chamber. A specimen chuck is likewise coated with cryoembedding medium. The medium changes from a clear, transparent appearance to opaque white as it begins to freeze.

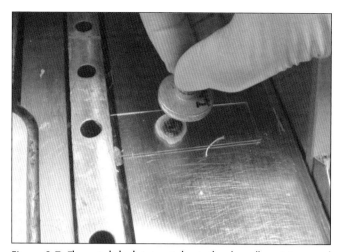

Figure 3.7. The coated chuck is inverted onto the glass-adherent tissue, and freezing is completed.

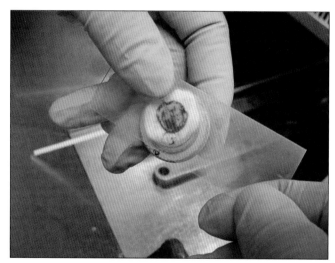

Figure 3.8. Running a warm finger across the glass surface will allow it to be removed from the block face. The result is a perfectly flat block face that requires no trimming.

The orientation requirements of the tissue sample during embedding may dictate which embedding method is used. When precise orientation is essential, the use of a metal mold may provide better precision than applying the specimen directly to a chuck coated with cryoembedding medium. Ensuring that the entire sample is in the same plane within the block is especially challenging when freezing the sample directly onto a chuck. This technique usually requires that the block be trimmed or faced before sections can be obtained.

A glass microscope slide can also be used as an embedding platform for freezing tissue.[4] This technique utilizes materials readily available in the laboratory and allows greater embedding precision, as the sample can be viewed from both sides of the glass while providing a perfectly flat and perpendicular block face, which eliminates the need for trimming or facing of the block prior

to sectioning. In this method, the tissue is placed directly onto the pre-chilled glass surface and arranged so that the face to be cut is touching the glass; the tissue will adhere to the glass and remain as placed. This method is illustrated in detail in Figures 3.5 through 3.8.

Regardless of the embedding method chosen, it is prudent to leave a border of cryoembedding medium around the tissue in order to provide a surface on which to apply a brush or other implement that can be used to "draw" the section down the knife surface as the blade passes through the block during sectioning.

Sample temperature will largely determine the ease with which a frozen tissue will section. In general, nonfatty tissues will section well between -15° and -20°C, while fatty tissues, such as breast, skin, adrenal, nervous tissue, etc, will section more easily when the sample is closer to -30°C. When sectioning difficulties are encoun-

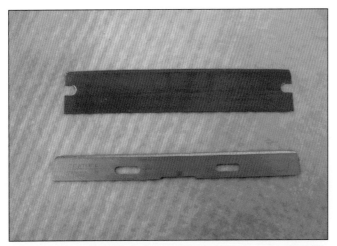

Figure 3.9. Disposable blades offer great convenience. The high-profile blade (top) is better suited for cryostat sectioning of dense frozen tissues.

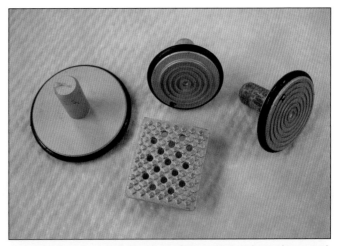

Figure 3.10. Cryostat chuck designs are often proprietary. The circular type with a post mount allows a specimen to be rotated a full 360 degrees, offering greater flexibility when sectioning. The rectangular type can likewise be rotated to one of four positions, each 90 degrees apart, to achieve a similar benefit for sectioning.

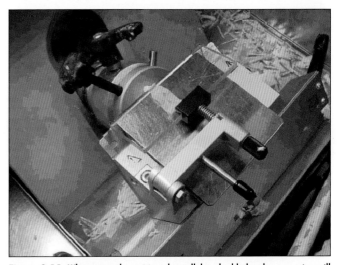

Figure 3.11. When properly positioned parallel to the blade edge, a section will glide smoothly beneath the anti-roll device.

tered and instrument problems have been ruled out, one can, through trial and error, alter the specimen temperature to observe sectioning characteristics. If a warmer block is desired, placing a gloved thumb against the block face momentarily will allow sufficient warming to determine if the sectioning characteristics of the tissue improve. Conversely, if the sample must be chilled further, commercially available refrigerant aerosol sprays or a metal heat extractor may be used for this purpose.

Sectioning with disposable microtome blades has become quite popular, as this approach offers a ready supply of sharp cutting edges, and the blades can be quickly brought to cryostat temperatures. Frozen tissue blocks are significantly harder than processed tissues as interstitial water has been frozen in the sample; therefore, if sectioning is not carried out with a conventional cryostat knife, high-profile disposable blades are needed to withstand the stresses of slicing through blocks of such firmness. Low-profile blades will likely contribute to sectioning artifacts resulting from blade flex and are not the best choice for cryostat sectioning (see Figure 3.9).

Most cryostat specimen chucks use a solid steel post to anchor the sample to the microtome (Figure 3.10). This design allows the specimen to be rotated, which can be very advantageous during sectioning. A specimen that does not section well often may need only to be rotated to a different plane to cure the problem. This is especially so if the sample is much longer in one plane than another. In general, the shortest path through the specimen is the easiest to section.

Cryostat manufacturers offer a variety of anti-roll devices that, when used properly, can be of great help in obtaining a flat section. These devices require a high degree of technical skill and are often more of a hindrance than a help. Frozen sections have a tendency to bunch up at the blade edge and often require manual manipulation. The anti-roll device can make sectioning stress free if properly positioned and aligned to the cutting edge. This allows the section to glide beneath the plate as the blade travels through the block face (Figure 3.11). The anti-roll device is not the best choice when cryostats are used by multiple individuals, as the device can easily become misaligned or damaged. As an alternative, skill in drawing the section along the blade with a cold camel's hair brush can be learned quickly and allows one to achieve high-quality sections rapidly (Figure 3.12).

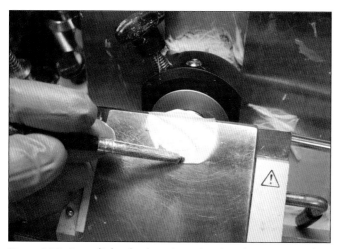

Figure 3.12. A camel's hair brush can be used to draw the section away from the blade edge to attain a flat section. This is a skill that can be learned quickly provided the brush bristles are kept clean and cold, and the blade holder surface is free of debris.

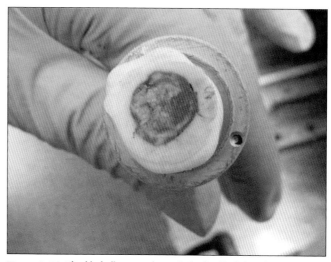

Figure 3.13. This block illustrates the goal of a flat block face that encompasses all of the tissue submitted.

Some manufacturers of modern cryostats have isolated the microtome from the freezer chamber, exposing only the chuck holder and tissue sample to the cold environment. This is especially beneficial, as it tends to avoid ice formation within the advance mechanism of the instrument. Ice formation is not uncommon in older cryostat models due to condensation of moisture from the air during cryostat operation. This may create a myriad of sectioning difficulties that can only be corrected with a time-consuming defrost, cleaning, and lubrication of the unit. Owners of older-generation units should be sensitive to keeping the window of the cryostat chamber closed whenever sectioning is not being performed in order to reduce the likelihood of condensation freezing within the microtome mechanism.

Controls

Blocks of fresh tissue from a large specimen that has been submitted for frozen section examination (eg, uterus, thyroid) can be frozen and maintained for several days in a temperature-controlled freezer or cryostat that does not have an automatic thaw-defrost cycle. Carefully wrapping the block in aluminum foil can retard the inevitable desiccation of the tissue and ice crystal artifact; when these become significant, the block must be discarded. A section of the control block should be prepared, stained, and examined with comparison to the previous day's slide on any day in which a frozen section is anticipated, prior to sectioning the current patient tissue, in order to assure that all aspects of the cryotomy and stain are performing optimally.

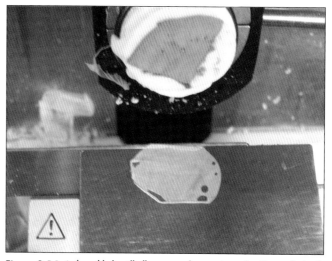

Figure 3.14. A sharp blade will allow a complete section to lay flat on the knife holder surface with minimal distortion.

What Should Be Seen in an Optimally Prepared Frozen Section

The optimal frozen section begins with an evenly and completely frozen tissue block in which the block face to be sectioned is flat and includes a complete, full-faced section of the tissue submitted; an optimal block face is illustrated in Figure 3.13. The section should be free of ice crystal artifact, knife lines, or tears and, if optimally prepared, should advance evenly onto the surface of the knife holder with minimal distortion (Figure 3.14). The H&E-stained frozen section should possess all of the tinctorial properties observed in paraffin sections, as described in detail in chapter 4 and illustrated in Figures 4.1 to 4.3.

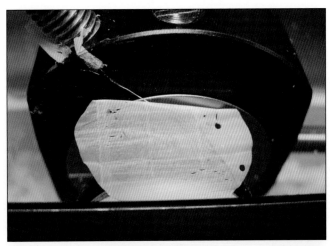

Figure 3.15. Debris on the knife edge will track through the section, damaging it. Careful cleaning of the knife edge, both front and back, may correct the problem if the cutting edge has not been damaged.

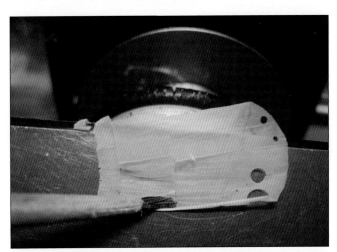

Figure 3.16. Damage to the cutting edge will cause tearing of the section in the direction of block travel through the blade. Slide the blade left or right in the blade holder to a new cutting surface to correct the problem.

Problems Encountered With the Frozen Section Technique

PROBLEM: The Section Shreds as it Comes Off the Knife

APPEARANCE: The section will exhibit visible knife lines (Figure 3.15), tears (Figures 3.16 and 3.17), or marked fragmentation (Figure 3.18).

CAUSES:
- The knife edge is damaged or contains debris.
- The tissue contains material(s) that will not section at this temperature.
- The tissue contains sutures, staples, or other foreign materials.

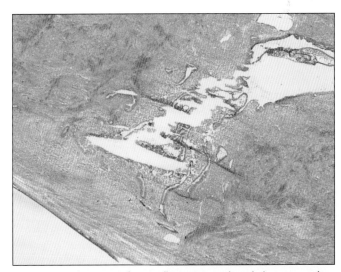

Figure 3.17. This section of uterus illustrates tears through the tissue resulting from debris on the blade edge or within the block.

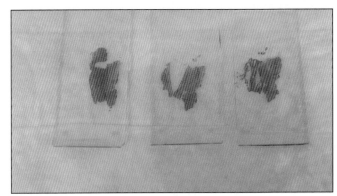

Figure 3.18. Defects or debris on the blade edge can cause shredding or other defects in the section.

SOLUTIONS:
- Clean the knife edge or replace the blade if necessary.
- Decrease or increase the block temperature.
- Remove foreign materials or prepare a new sample free of such materials.

PROBLEM: The Section Bunches Up at the Knife Edge or Does Not Slide Off the Knife Edge Smoothly

APPEARANCE: The section folds upon itself or rolls up immediately behind the knife edge and cannot be flattened by a brush or anti-roll device (Figure 3.19).

CAUSES:
- The blade holder surface is dirty or iced up.
- The blade surface is too warm.
- The knife angle is incorrect.
- The blade is dull.

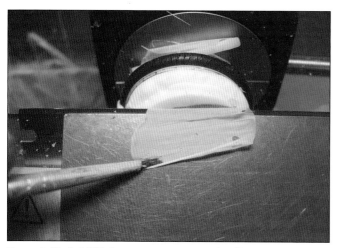

Figure 3.19. A dull blade or improper cutting angle will cause compression of the section.

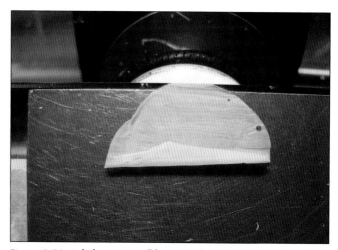

Figure 3.20. A thicker section will have a tendency to curl on the blade holder surface. In this instance, a dull blade will not slice cleanly, creating a thicker section that will be followed by a section that is too thin (see Figure 3.21).

SOLUTIONS:

- Clean the blade holder with alcohol to remove ice or debris.
- Cool the blade.
- Adjust the blade angle to the correct setting.
- Try a different cutting edge of the blade by moving the blade (left/right), or replace the blade.

PROBLEM: One Section Is Thick and the Next Is Thin or Incomplete, or There are Thick and Thin Areas Within the Same Section

APPEARANCE: A thick section is opaque and often curls on the surface of the blade holder (Figure 3.20). A thin section tears and/or fragments easily as it advance from the knife edge (Figure 3.21).

CAUSES:

- The blade is loose.
- The blade holder is loose.
- The block is loose.
- The blade is dull.
- The microtome is not advancing properly.

SOLUTIONS:

- Verify that the blade is clamped down tightly. If not, secure the blade. If it is tightly clamped, then the blade holder may require cleaning to remove debris that has accumulated within the holder, preventing a firm hold on the blade.
- Verify that the blade holder is tightly clamped to the microtome base.

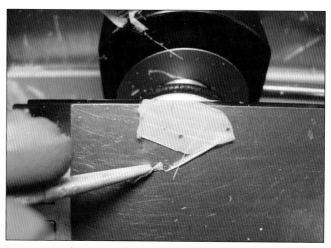

Figure 3.21. This section is fragile because it is too thin, following the thicker section in Figure 3.20, obtained with a dull cutting edge.

- Confirm that the chuck is clamped tightly in the microtome; if it is, embedding medium may be poorly adhered to the chuck. If necessary the block can be adhered to a new chuck with embedding medium.
- Replace the blade. A dull blade will chop through the block, rather than slice cleanly. This can create a thick section, leaving less or little tissue for the next rotation of the microtome.
- Defrost, disinfect, thoroughly dry, and lubricate the instrument. In most instances, this will solve advancing difficulties; if not, a service call may be needed.

PROBLEM: The Section Is Incomplete; Portions of the Tissue Block Do Not Section

APPEARANCE: The tissue exhibits multiple micro-tears parallel to the knife edge, which easily fragment, and portions of tissue visible in the block are not represented on the tissue section (Figure 3.22).

CAUSES:

- The cryostat temperature is incorrect for the tissue being sectioned.
- The blade edge is dull or contains debris.

SOLUTIONS:

- Change the block temperature. Some tissue components, like fat or other lipid-rich tissues, will require much colder temperatures in order to section properly. Aerosol refrigerant sprays may be utilized to make the block face colder. A gloved finger held against the block face momentarily can elevate the temperature. Some trial and error may be necessary to find the optimal cutting temperature for that specimen.
- Clean the blade edge, including the back edge, where debris may have accumulated; replace the blade if necessary.

PROBLEM: The Block Falls Off the Chuck While Sectioning

APPEARANCE: When the block is being faced, the majority of the tissue block containing the tissue abruptly "pops off" the surface, leaving behind the chuck and a thin layer of residual embedding medium.

CAUSE:

- The embedding medium was not properly adhered to the chuck.

SOLUTIONS:

- Re-adhere the tissue block by applying embedding medium to a clean chuck, and allow the block to freeze completely before sectioning is attempted.
- Never store chucks with adherent embedding medium in the cryostat overnight; the defrost cycle will compromise adherence and contribute to this problem.

PROBLEM: Tissue Chips Out of the Block During Block Trimming or Sectioning

APPEARANCE: The tissue block remains adherent to the chuck; however, the tissue fractures while the block is being faced, and a portion of the tissue detaches from the remainder of the block face, leaving a visible defect.

CAUSES:

- Rapid advancement of the microtome during aggressive rough trimming.

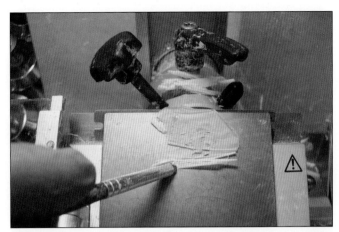

Figure 3.22. Incorrect temperature will cause sectioning difficulties, including an incomplete section.

- The tissue may be too hard for the embedding medium to hold and is unsuitable for frozen sections.
- A loose blade or tissue block, causing erratic movement of the knife through the tissue.
- Erratic advancement of the microtome.
- Freezing at extremely low temperatures (eg, isopentane in liquid nitrogen) and not allowing the block to come to chamber temperature.

SOLUTIONS:

- The block should be advanced in small increments, especially with very dense tissues.
- Very dense tissues may be unsuitable for frozen sections.
- Verify that the blade and block are secure, tightening all instrument settings.
- The microtome may require defrosting and lubrication due to ice formation in the mechanism. Defrost, clean, and thoroughly dry the microtome before lubricating. Any remaining moisture in the advance mechanism will re-freeze at cryostat temperatures.
- Allow the block to come to cryostat temperature before attempting the section.

References

1. Callis G. Preparation and snap freezing of murine tissues for research immunohistochemistry and routine hematoxylin & eosin staining. *HistoLogic.* 2004;37:4-7.
2. Bancroft JD, Gamble M. *Theory and Practice of Histological Techniques.* 5th ed. New York, NY: Churchill Livingstone; 2002: 101.
3. Peters SR. The art of embedding tissue for frozen section, part II: frozen block cryoembedding. *J Histotechnol.* 2003;26:23-28.
4. Geddis C. A novel technique to embed tissues for frozen section cryotomy. *HistoLogic.* 2004;37:7-10.

Hematoxylin and Eosin

Sue E. Lewis

The hematoxylin and eosin (H&E) stain is the primary diagnostic stain used in the practice of anatomic pathology. H&E staining permits assessment of the general relationship among cells, allowing the basic architectural elements of epithelial, connective, nervous, and muscle tissues to be demonstrated. Simply defined, hematoxylin should stain nuclear cellular elements, whereas eosin should stain cytoplasmic cellular elements.

It is important to recognize the effects that tissue-grossing practices, fixation, and processing have on routine H&E staining. Careful and scientific control of all possible factors within the staining procedure itself can eliminate many problems; however, the H&E stain is only as good as the grossing, fixation, and processing steps that prepare the tissue section for the staining sequence. In addition, the final procedural steps of dehydration, clearing, and coverslipping are equally important in producing an excellent H&E slide.

Hematoxylin "staining" is actually a misnomer. Hematoxylin is extracted from the Central American logwood tree, and the hematoxylin dye (powder) is classified as a flavone, a type of pigment. It does not have the ability to stain anything because it is colorless and has no ability to bind to tissues. It is only after the oxidation of the hematoxylin dye that a colored product, hematein, is formed. Hematein is the active ingredient in the hematoxylin solution. The hematoxylin solutions routinely used in the laboratory are a combination of hematein (oxidized hematoxylin) and a metal mordant. Formulations of hematoxylin solutions vary in the (1) oxidizer, (2) mordant, (3) proportion of the mordant to hematoxylin dye, and (4) addition of acid, stabilizers, or preservatives.

The staining specificity of hematoxylin solutions is achieved through tight control of the solution's pH. Optimal hematoxylin solutions have a pH of approximately 2.5. Daily pH monitoring of the laboratory's hematoxylin solution can help prevent fluctuations in staining quality. The most common reasons for pH shift include the inadvertent carryover of distilled or tap water from slide rinses before staining, and the unavoidable progressive oxidation that occurs when the staining solution is exposed to light and air.

Hematoxylin staining may be carried out through progressive or regressive staining methods. Progressive hematoxylin solutions deposit the stain primarily in the cell nuclei and only minimally in the cytoplasm. Therefore, progressive staining does not require subsequent acidic differentiation (see below). The most commonly used progressive hematoxylin stains include Gill and Mayer. In contrast, the most frequently used regressive stains include Harris, Delafield, and Ehrlich. Regressive staining requires that the tissue section first be overstained with hematoxylin. The excess dye is then removed in a very controlled manner. The process of selectively removing excess dye is called *differentiation*. Differentiation is most commonly accomplished using a weak solution of acid, followed by extensive rinses in either distilled or tap water. When differentiation is optimally performed with an alum-hematoxylin solution, nuclear chromatin should be dark purple, with the nuclear membrane appearing as a purple ring. The well-differentiated stain is often described as "crisp," which can also be defined as exhibiting high contrast between the purple-staining nuclear chromatin and the colorless or pale-staining nucleoplasm.

Bluing of the hematoxylin-stained and differentiated tissue section is the final step related to nuclear staining. It is critical that the bluing agent be completely removed. Thorough washing in water is required, because any residual alkalinity in the tissue sections will prevent eosin from binding during the next step. Also, residual bluing solution can influence the intensity and quality of the eosin stain.

Eosin and phloxine are xanthene dyes often used as counterstains in the H&E procedure. Eosin, an anionic dye, is used most commonly. As a counterstain in the H&E procedure, eosin should never overwhelm or obscure the nuclear staining.

Collagen, smooth muscle, and erythrocytes should exhibit three distinct and different shades of pink. When eosin is properly differentiated, the pathologist is able to distinguish the cytoplasm of different cell types and the different types of connective tissue. Red blood cells and other intensely eosinophilic structures (eg, Paneth cell

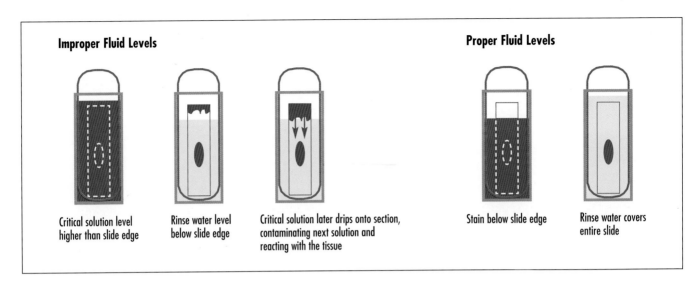

Improper Fluid Levels

Critical solution level higher than slide edge

Rinse water level below slide edge

Critical solution later drips onto section, contaminating next solution and reacting with the tissue

Proper Fluid Levels

Stain below slide edge

Rinse water covers entire slide

granules) should always be a richer, brighter, or more intense red than other structures. Cell cytoplasm and muscle fibers should differ from collagen, and both should be less brilliant than the red blood cells. Whether the collagen or the cytoplasm/muscle is the intermediate pink color is determined by many factors, such as the type and duration of fixation, the degree of heating and drying, the formulation of the stain, the differentiation step after the eosin, and the structure of the collagen itself. In any case, the two tissue elements—cell cytoplasm/muscle fibers and collagen—should appear different shades of pink.

The two most common forms of eosin dye include eosin B (blue) and eosin Y (yellow). Eosin Y is available as either an aqueous or alcoholic solution. The best staining with eosin occurs at a pH of 4.0 to 4.5. If a more intense eosin counterstain is preferred, a combination of eosin and phloxine B can be used, which gives a very vivid spectrum of pinks. Eosin staining also involves overstaining of the tissue section, similar to that of hematoxylin. Therefore, it also requires a differentiation step employing either alcohol, when using an alcoholic eosin, or water, when using an aqueous eosin solution. The most common problems encountered with eosin staining are related to pH shift or solution depletion from too many slides having been stained. Some laboratories successfully extend the viability of their stain by continuously adjusting the pH into the 4.0 to 4.5 range.

It is important to watch the fluid levels of rinse solutions during the H&E procedure. If a solution is not completely rinsed off, it can drip down onto the tissue or continue to react. For example, incomplete rinsing after acid-alcohol will allow the acid to continue removing hematoxylin, resulting in lighter nuclear staining. The

fluid levels of critical solutions, including stains, differentiator, and bluing solution, should be high enough to just barely cover the slides. In contrast, the fluid level for the water rinse/wash steps should be high. With automatic stainers, flow rates must be adjusted to completely rinse the slides of the previous reagent (ie, the water rinse after hematoxylin should be free of any blue color when the slides leave that station).

Controls

Routine daily use of a multi-tissue control block to assess and document the quality of the H&E stain can be a valuable tool for troubleshooting staining problems. A control block containing well-fixed and optimally processed tissue helps to identify whether the cause of a staining problem is processing or staining. General recommendations for types of tissues to be included in a control block include artery, a small piece of gastrointestinal tract, cerebellum, spleen, and placenta. Each day, a section should be cut from the control block and stained, then compared to the stained control slide from the previous day. Color intensity and stain specificity should be equal and consistent. Microscopic examination of these varied tissues allows evaluation for optimal nuclear staining (as determined by well-defined nuclear membranes; an admixture of open, crisp blue and dense, closed chromatin patterns; and acidophilic nucleoli), while the three-tone effect of the eosin counterstain is evaluated by looking at erythrocytes, smooth muscle, and collagen. Whenever a tissue section shows both correct and incorrect staining patterns, the fault is in the fixation or in the processing of the specimen. Correct staining in selected areas of a tissue section could not have occurred if there had been a staining error.

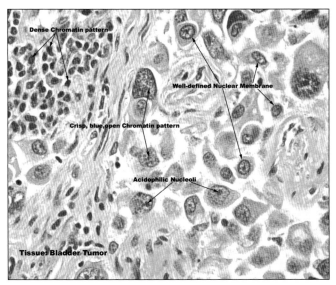

Figure 4.1. This section of a carcinoma exhibits excellent nuclear detail. Note the dense chromatin pattern of the smaller lymphocytes and the acidophilic nucleoli, well-defined nuclear membranes, and crisp blue, open chromatin patterns of the large tumor cells.

What Should Be Seen in an Optimal H&E Stain

Nuclei should show a variety of crisp, blue chromatin patterns and a well-defined blue nuclear membrane. There should not be any nuclear defects such as smudginess, bubbling, or paleness. There should be no cell shrinkage or unusual spaces between cells. Figure 4.1 shows excellent nuclear detail. Note the different nuclear patterns demonstrated: dense chromatin staining of lymphocytes, acidophilic nucleoli, well-defined nuclear membranes, and crisp blue, open chromatin in the epithelioid cells. Figure 4.2 is an excellent example of the nuclear detail expected when lymphoid tissue is stained with H&E. Most tissue sections should demonstrate three distinct shades of eosin, with the cell cytoplasm, smooth muscle, collagen, and red blood cells showing characteristic stain intensities. Figure 4.3 illustrates optimal tri-tonal eosin staining in a section of uterus. Note how the smooth muscle and collagen contrast with each other, while the red blood cells show a brighter shade of eosin. The section should be coverslipped so that the mounting medium covers the entire area under the coverslip, with no mounting medium on top of the coverslip.

There are a number of challenges to producing a high-quality H&E stain in the laboratory. Table 4.1 gives the most common staining problems identified in the first four NSH/CAP HistoQIP Program (HQIP) challenges.

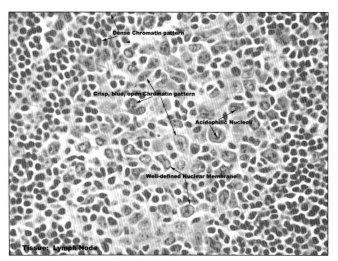

Figure 4.2. This section of lymph node demonstrates the typical range of nuclear staining. The smaller lymphocytes show condensed chromatin, while the larger lymphoid cells show an open chromatin pattern, crisp nuclear membranes, and acidophilic nucleoli.

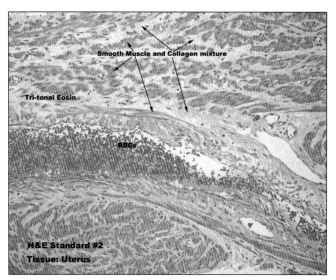

Figure 4.3. This section of uterus demonstrates tri-tonal eosin staining. The smooth muscle and collagen show two distinct shades; the red blood cells show brighter eosin staining.

All data are expressed as a percentage of that staining problem seen in the total number of slides submitted for each tissue. Among the other problems seen in the HQIP Program slides, but not listed in the table, are uneven staining, mounting artifact, and stain precipitate. Each one of these problems is specifically addressed in this chapter.

Table 4.1. The Most Common Staining Problems in the First Four HQIP H&E Challenges

Tissue H&E	% Nuclei Not Crisp/Smudgy Nuclei/No Chromatin Pattern	% Only 1 or 2 Shades of Cytoplasmic Stain	% Poor Contrast	% Cytoplasmic Stain Too Dark	% Nuclear Stain Too Dark	% Cytoplasmic Stain Too Light	% Nuclear Stain Too Light
Breast	23.7	28.7	17.8	7.3	7.9	7.9	7.6
Skin	20.2	23.0	20.8	8.0	4.4	5.3	11.9
Lymph Node	24.2	40.0	17.0	10.7	13.4	8.3	1.0
Lung	25.3	29.0	16.7	15.5	5.6	6.1	2.9
Uterus	22.1	35.8	14.0	4.4	2.6	6.2	3.8
Colon	30.0	22.3	13.0	3.7	3.5	6.5	3.5
Bone Marrow	42.5	12.8	13.8	8.1	17.9	2.5	2.4
Liver	39.7	31.3	20.4	9.3	5.0	4.7	6.8
Average	**28.5**	**27.9**	**16.7**	**8.4**	**7.5**	**5.4**	**5.0**

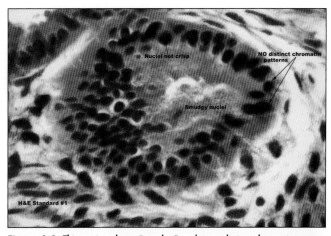

Figure 4.4. This section shows "smudgy" nuclei; no distinct chromatin pattern is observed.

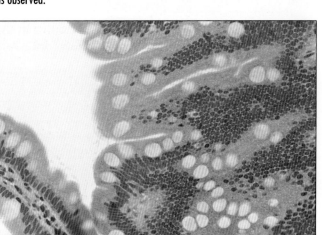

Figure 4.5. In this section of small intestine, the nuclei appear as "blue blobs," lacking distinct chromatin patterns.

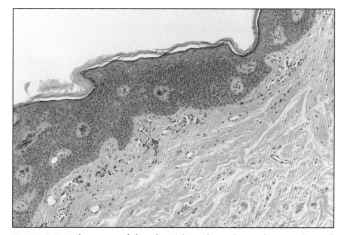

Figure 4.6. In this section of skin, the nuclei in the epidermis show no cell-to-cell variation in chromatin pattern when viewed at low magnification.

Problems Encountered With the H&E Stain

PROBLEM: Nuclei Not Crisp, "Smudgy" Nuclei, Nuclear Bubbling, or No Distinct Chromatin Patterns

APPEARANCE: The nuclear chromatin is not sharply defined (smudgy nuclei). There is no variation in nuclear chromatin patterns among cells, and there is no variation in chromatin staining within one nucleus (Figures 4.4, 4,5, and 4.6).

CAUSES:

- Fixation is poor or incomplete.
- Water was not completely removed during dehydration and clearing.

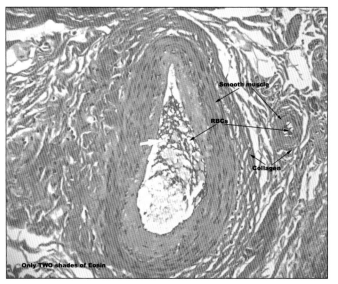

Figure 4.7. In this section of connective tissue containing a muscular artery, note that there are only two shades of eosin. Smooth muscle and collagen exhibit similar staining.

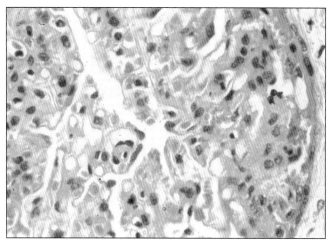

Figure 4.8. This kidney glomerulus shows only two shades of eosin. Only the red blood cells are differentially stained.

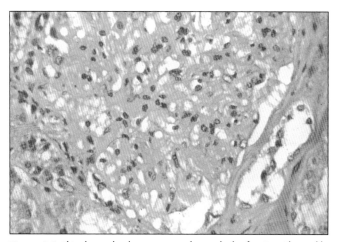

Figure 4.9. This glomerulus demonstrates only one shade of eosin, with an additional problem of improper ("smudgy") nuclear staining.

- Slides were exposed to excessive heat during processing or drying.

SOLUTIONS:

- Allow tissues to fix for a longer time; use stir plates to circulate the fixative in cassette-holding containers; exchange the fixative in the cassette-holding containers at regular intervals throughout the workday.

- Ensure that the dehydration and clearing are complete by reviewing timed steps in each solution; ensure that solutions are rotated and/or changed on a schedule to prevent solution exhaustion.

- Ensure that tissues are exposed to high temperatures for as short a time as possible, and use temperatures only as high as absolutely necessary; assess whether paraffin baths may elevate retort temperatures during dehydration and clearing steps, and adjust times accordingly to eliminate excessive heat.

- Stand slides containing cut sections on end or on edge and allow them to drain thoroughly before drying at as low a temperature as possible. Do not exceed 70°C.

PROBLEM: Three Shades of Eosin Not Seen

APPEARANCE: Only one or two shades of eosin can be seen (Figures 4.7, 4.8, and 4.9).

CAUSES:

- Fixation is inadequate.
- Improper processing occurred.
- There is poor differentiation of the eosin.
- Eosin solution is not at the correct pH.

SOLUTIONS:

- Ensure adequate fixation by prolonging the time allowed; use stir plates to circulate the fixative in cassette-holding containers; exchange the fixative in the cassette-holding containers at regular intervals throughout the workday.

- Ensure that proper processing occurs: all water must be removed during dehydration and clearing; validate timed steps in all solutions for completeness.

- Ensure good differentiation of the eosin. Differentiation occurs best in 70% alcohol solutions and to a lesser extent in higher-percentage alcohols; therefore, adding a 70% alcohol to the series or increasing the time in 70% alcohol will aid in differentiation. Ensure that the 70% alcohol used in the differentiation step is changed at regular intervals.

- Ensure that the pH of the eosin is between 4.0 and 4.5.

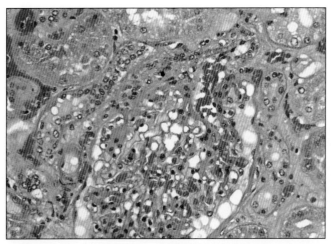

Figure 4.10. There is very poor contrast between the hematoxylin and eosin in this section of kidney; only two shades of eosin are observed.

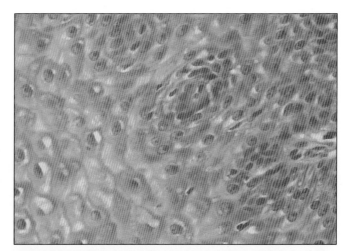

Figure 4.12. In this high-magnification view of squamous epithelium, all tissue elements are stained various shades of pink, with virtually no contrast between nucleus and cytoplasm.

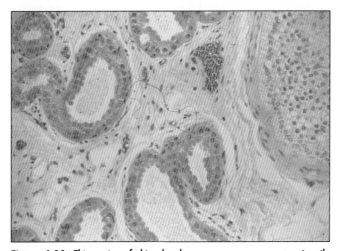

Figure 4.11. This section of skin also demonstrates poor contrast, primarily because of the pale staining of the nuclei.

PROBLEM: Poor Contrast

APPEARANCE: The nuclear stain is partially masked by the cytoplasmic stain (Figures 4.10, 4.11, and 4.12).

CAUSES:

- The nuclear stain is too dark for the cytoplasmic stain.
- The nuclear stain is too pale for the cytoplasmic stain.
- The cytoplasmic stain is too dark for the nuclear stain.
- The cytoplasmic stain is too pale for the nuclear stain.

SOLUTIONS:

- To decrease the intensity of the hematoxylin staining, decrease the time in the hematoxylin solution or increase the time in the differentiating solution. Check the pH of the hematoxylin daily to maintain an optimally acidic solution (pH 2.5 ± 0.2). Adjust the pH using the acid included in the original formulation.
- To increase the intensity of the hematoxylin stain,

increase the time in the hematoxylin solution or decrease the time in the differentiating solution.

- Ensure that water rinses are thorough, and exert enough force (pounds per square inch) to remove all excess stain.
- Water pH can be affected by agricultural runoff or other contaminants. Monitor the water for fluctuations in pH.
- To decrease the intensity of the cytoplasmic stain, decrease the time in the stain, dilute the stain, allow more time in 70% alcohol, or use 50% alcohol for differentiation.
- To increase the intensity of the cytoplasmic stain, increase the time in the stain, allow a longer time in the stain, or decrease the time in lower percentage alcohols. Check the pH of the eosin; it should be between 4.0 and 4.5.

PROBLEM: Cytoplasmic Stain Is Too Dark

APPEARANCE: The cytoplasmic stain is so intense that the differentiation between collagen, smooth muscle, and red cells is lost (Figures 4.13 and 4.14). The nuclei begin to show staining with eosin as well as with the hematoxylin. Nucleoli, if present, should be distinctly acidophilic (eosinophilic) in a well-stained section; this is *not* an attribute of "cytoplasmic stain is too dark."

CAUSES:

- Exposure of sections to the eosin solution is prolonged.
- There is inadequate eosin differentiation in the alcohols that follow the eosin stain; aqueous formulations stain tissue darker than alcohol-based stains.
- The alcohol rinse is not performed properly after the eosin stain.

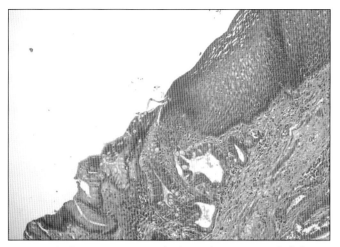

Figure 4.13. This tissue section stained with H&E shows an extremely dark counterstain, which obscures hematoxylin staining in the cell nuclei.

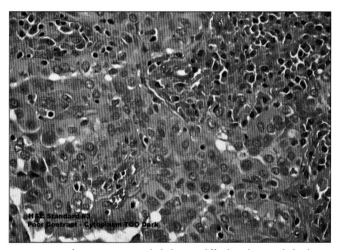

Figure 4.14. The eosin stain is so dark that it is difficult to distinguish the densely acidophilic tissue elements.

- Eosin may be too concentrated, especially if phloxine is present.
- If using an alcoholic eosin product, water contamination may have interfered with complete differentiation.
- Isopropyl alcohol was used as the dehydrating solution; isopropyl alcohol does not differentiate eosin within tissue sections in the same manner as ethyl alcohol.

SOLUTIONS:
- Decrease the time in the eosin solution.
- Increase the time in the dehydrating alcohols.
- Change the first alcohol from 100% to 95% alcohol or from 95% to 70% alcohol.
- Change to another eosin formulation (eg, aqueous or alcoholic formulation).
- If phloxine is present, decrease the concentration or change to an eosin-only formulation.
- Change the type of alcohol used.

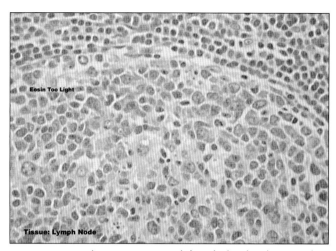

Figure 4.15. Cytoplasmic staining is very light in this lymph node section; three distinct shades of eosin cannot be identified.

PROBLEM: Cytoplasmic Stain Is Too Light

APPEARANCE: The cytoplasmic stain is light and does not optimally demonstrate three distinct colors of eosin (Figure 4.15). The cytoplasmic stain does not contrast well with the nuclear stain.

CAUSES:
- The eosin solution is exhausted.
- The pH of the eosin staining solution is greater than 4.5.
- The bluing solution is not completely washed out before the slides are transferred to the eosin solution.
- The differentiation in diluted alcohols is prolonged.
- The alcohol rinse after the eosin stain is incorrectly performed.
- The staining time in eosin is too brief.

SOLUTIONS:
- Replace the old eosin solution with a fresh eosin solution.
- Check the pH of the staining solution; it should be between 4.0 and 4.5. If necessary, adjust the pH with concentrated acetic acid.
- Give slides a longer rinse in running water (or more changes) after the bluing solution. Carryover of bluing reagent can raise the pH of the eosin or actually destain the eosin in the tissue section.
- Decrease the time in dilute alcohols after the eosin step.
- Change the alcohol rinse to anhydrous alcohol, or, if using 70% alcohol, change to 95%.
- Increase the staining time in eosin solution.

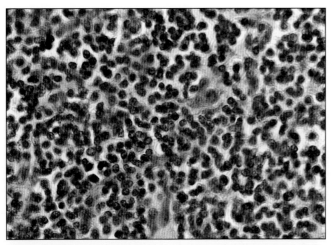

Figure 4.16. The lymphocyte nuclei in this section of lymph node are darkly stained, obscuring the internal nuclear detail. The overstaining with hematoxylin is accentuated by the poor tissue processing and the excessive thickness of the section.

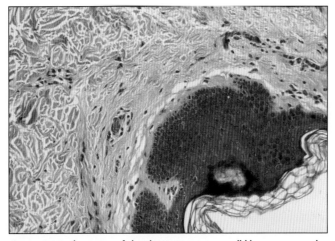

Figure 4.17. This section of skin demonstrates an overall blue appearance due to excessive hematoxylin staining, with loss of nuclear detail and a lack of eosin differentiation.

PROBLEM: Nuclear Stain Is Too Dark

APPEARANCE: The nuclear stain is so dark that the chromatin pattern is lost and some nonnuclear elements show hematoxylin staining (Figures 4.16 and 4.17). When evaluating the hematoxylin stain, note that blue staining of goblet cells and mucin is not an artifact but is due to the hematoxylin formulation used (eg, Gill).

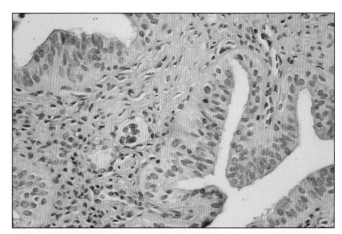

Figure 4.18. This section of cervix shows incomplete deparaffinization, resulting in a light hematoxylin stain and smudgy nuclei. The nuclei are homogenous and pale throughout the section, with no distinct differentiation of nuclear chromatin.

CAUSES:
- The hematoxylin solution is too concentrated.
- Too much time is allowed in the hematoxylin solution.
- There is inadequate differentiation of the hematoxylin stain.
- The pH of the hematoxylin solution is incorrect.

SOLUTIONS:
- Dilute the hematoxylin with water or glycerin.
- Decrease the time allowed in hematoxylin.
- Allow more time in the differentiating solution.
- Check the pH of the hematoxylin solution; most hematoxylin solutions require a pH of approximately 2.5.

PROBLEM: Nuclear Stain Is Too Light

APPEARANCE: The nuclear stain is so light that well-defined chromatin patterns cannot be seen (Figure 4.18).

CAUSES:
- There is incomplete deparaffinization.
- The hematoxylin solution is exhausted or used beyond its shelf life.
- The hematoxylin solution is diluted by carryover from a previous water rinse.
- Sections are overdifferentiated by using overly concentrated acid-alcohol solutions, or the sections remain too long in the acid-alcohol.
- The staining time is too short in the hematoxylin solution.

- Tap water is used in the water rinses before and after staining. Tap water with a high concentration of iron, chlorine, or sulfur can act as excess mordant or differentiator and actually destain hematoxylin. Use deionized or distilled water for rinsing.
- Poor fixation and/or processing, resulting in tissues that are unable to bind stain.

SOLUTIONS:

- Increase the number of changes of the xylene, or xylene substitute, used for removal of paraffin.
- Increase the amount of time in each xylene, or xylene substitute, used for removal of paraffin.
- Change to a fresh hematoxylin solution.
- Decrease the time in the differentiating solution, or dilute the differentiating solution.
- Increase the time in the hematoxylin solution.
- Ensure thorough water rinsing of stained sections.
- Ensure that the sections are well dehydrated and cleared during processing.

PROBLEM: Uneven Eosin or Hematoxylin Staining

APPEARANCE: The stain varies in intensity in different areas of the section. Uneven eosin staining is most commonly observed; however, uneven hematoxylin staining may occur as well (Figures 4.19 and 4.20).

CAUSES:

- The section may be thick and thin.
- Some solutions are not high enough to cover the entire slide.
- The water rinse was not adequate after hematoxylin staining.
- The water rinse was not adequate after acid-alcohol, which is necessary to stop decolorization.
- The water rinse was not adequate after bluing.
- The alcohol rinse (dehydration) was not adequate after eosin staining.

SOLUTIONS:

- Recut the section, ensuring that it is of uniform thickness.
- Ensure that all solutions completely cover the slides.
- Increase the time and/or fluid level of the water rinses.

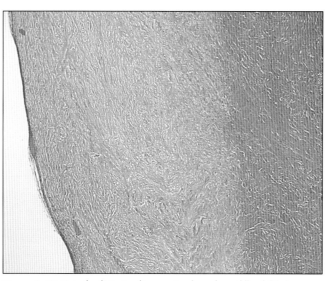

Figure 4.19. Note the distinctive line running down the middle of this tissue section. Part of this section demonstrates an overall red appearance that obscures the nuclear detail. This inconsistent staining is most likely due to an improper fluid level.

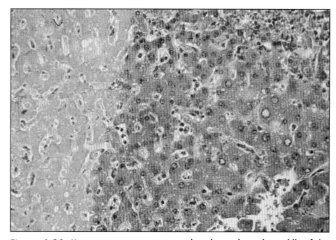

Figure 4.20. Uneven staining appears as a line drawn down the middle of this section of liver, which may be due to a low level of the hematoxylin solution.

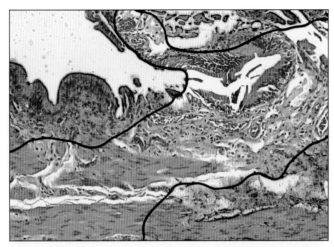

Figure 4.21. Note the obvious and uneven dark line throughout this tissue section, which is caused by evaporation of the mounting medium and the presence of air on part of the tissue.

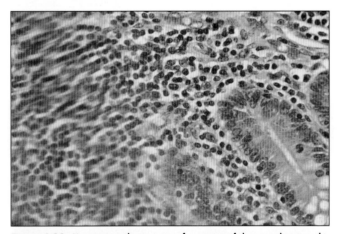

Figure 4.22. Mounting medium on top of a portion of the coverslip gives this tissue section a hazy appearance.

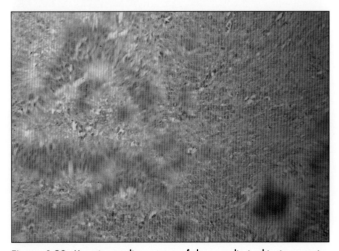

Figure 4.23. Mounting medium on top of the coverslip in this tissue section obscures the tissue morphology.

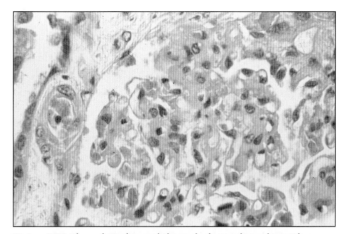

Figure 4.24. The nuclei in this renal glomerulus have a distinct brownish appearance, rather than the preferred blue-violet or blue-black.

PROBLEM: Mounting Artifact

APPEARANCE: Air is present under the coverslip and the microscopic image of the tissue is obscured (Figure 4.21), or mounting medium is present on top of the coverslip, making focusing on some areas of the tissue difficult (Figures 4.22 and 4.23).

CAUSES:

- The mounting medium has retracted from the edges of the coverslip.
- Air bubbles are trapped under the coverslip.
- There is mounting medium on top of the coverslip.

SOLUTIONS:

- Ensure that the mounting medium is neither too thick nor too thin.
- Change to fresh mounting medium.
- Ensure that air bubbles are not trapped under the coverslip.
- Ensure that mounting medium is not present on top of the coverslip.

PROBLEM: Red-Brown Nuclei

APPEARANCE: The nuclear stain has a distinct red-brown or reddish hue, often seen throughout the entire slide. Focusing up and down may also demonstrate various hues of red and brown (Figure 4.24).

CAUSES:

- The sections have not been sufficiently blued.
- The hematoxylin is breaking down.

SOLUTIONS:

- Increase the amount of time the sections remain in the bluing solution.

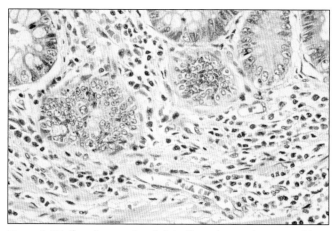

Figure 4.25. The collagen and epithelial cell cytoplasm in this section of large bowel have a bluish hue. There is also nuclear bubbling artifact.

- Change to a fresh solution of hematoxylin or to a different commercial supply.
- If using a programmable automated stainer, allow slides to have an initial rinse in a water wash station, then have them move to a second "clean" water wash station for thorough rinsing.
- Ensure that sections are thoroughly rinsed in water after both the hematoxylin and the bluing steps.

PROBLEM: Blue (Instead of Various Shades of Pink) Staining of Cellular Elements Such as Collagen or Smooth Muscle

APPEARANCE: Collagen, smooth muscle, and epithelial cytoplasm are a very light blue (Figure 4.25).

CAUSES:
- The pH of the hematoxylin solution is greater than 3.0.
- There was inadequate differentiation.
- Slides have spent too much time in the dehydrating/differentiation alcohols.
- The eosin is contaminated by carryover from the bluing solution.
- The acid-alcohol is too weak.
- The amount of time spent in acid-alcohol is too short.
- The hematoxylin stain formulation is not selective enough.

SOLUTIONS:
- Check the hematoxylin pH and adjust accordingly with acetic acid. Optimal pH should be 2.5; if using a commercially prepared hematoxylin solution, check with the manufacturer for their recommended pH range.

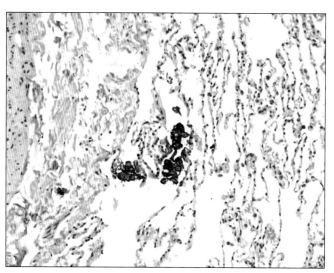

Figure 4.26. This section of lung tissue contains a large, dark purple aggregate of hematein precipitate.

- Increase the concentration of acid-alcohol.
- Increase the time spent in acid-alcohol.
- Increase the time spent in the water wash.
- Consider changing hematoxylin to a different formulation or obtaining from a different commercial supplier.

PROBLEM: Dark Precipitate Scattered Throughout the Section

APPEARANCE: Blue-black or purple precipitate is present on parts of the section (Figure 4.26).

CAUSES:
- Deteriorated hematoxylin (hematoxylin used beyond the expiration date or damaged from improper storage conditions) will show precipitate. Discard the solution and use new hematoxylin.
- Some hematoxylins form a metallic film on the surface of the solution. If the hematoxylin is not filtered before use, the metallic film transfers or adheres to the surface of the tissue section.

SOLUTIONS:
- Filter the hematoxylin solution daily before staining slides.
- Monitor the hematoxylin solution throughout the day for the appearance of a metallic sheen (hematein). If this is observed, either refilter or replace the hematoxylin.
- Ensure proper storage of hematoxylin solutions, according to manufacturer's guidelines.

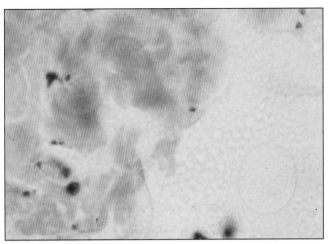

Figure 4.27. This high-magnification view illustrates water bubbles beneath the coverslip, obscuring the tissue morphology. This problem is due to incomplete dehydration of the section after staining.

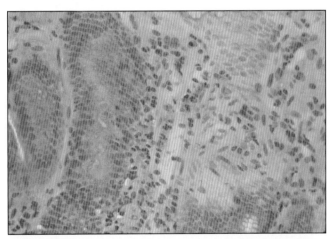

Figure 4.28. This gastrointestinal biopsy specimen has a diffusely hazy appearance, diminishing both the contrast and the nuclear detail. This problem is probably due to contamination of the dehydration or clearing solutions with water.

PROBLEM: Bubbles on the Tissue Section or in Tissue Spaces, Decreasing Clarity of the Section

APPEARANCE: Water bubbles are seen during microscopic examination of the section; the section has also lost its clarity (Figure 4.27).

CAUSE:

• The section is not completely dehydrated.

SOLUTION:

• Remove the coverslip and back the sections up to water. Repeat the dehydration steps with fresh solutions of alcohol and xylene.

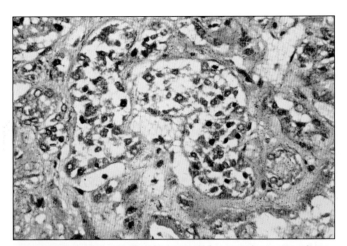

Figure 4.29. This slide was allowed to air-dry before coverslipping. Note the stippling in the cell nuclei.

PROBLEM: Sections With an Overall Hazy Appearance, or Eosin Bleeding Throughout the Section

APPEARANCE: The tissue appears hazy or out of focus when examined microscopically (Figure 4.28).

CAUSES:

• Solutions are contaminated with water from the previous solution.

• Sections were not adequately dehydrated after eosin staining.

SOLUTIONS:

• Design and implement a standardized, routine, solution change schedule for alcohols and xylenes that helps keep carryover from prior solutions to a minimum.

• Use a minimum of three changes of anhydrous alcohol, with 1 minute per change at the end of the staining series.

• Increase the number of stations of anhydrous alcohol or the amount of time per station at the end of the series.

COMMENT: Alcohol can absorb moisture from the air, and the final alcohol then becomes contaminated, especially during humid weather. Xylene has the ability to bind small concentrations of water, but xylene substitutes cannot. Some "no water tolerance" xylene substitutes will therefore exhibit eosin bleeding. Consider using a drying agent in the anhydrous alcohols. To assess for water contamination, do a visual inspection of the staining solutions. The solutions may have a cloudy appearance or may have particles floating in them; alternately, the alcohols or xylenes turn "milky" at the beginning or the end of the series. It is important to know, however, that alcohol solutions can also appear completely clear when they are actually contaminated with water.

PROBLEM: Brown "Pigment" Throughout the Section, and Glossy Black Nuclei

APPEARANCE: The nuclei are black and refractile with brown stippling. A brown granular deposit, similar in appearance to formalin pigment, is sometimes seen throughout the section (Figure 4.29).

CAUSE:

• The tissue section dried out before the coverslip was applied.

SOLUTION:

• Remove the coverslip, take the slide back to water and allow it to stand for several minutes. Then dehydrate, clear, and remount the slide with mounting medium and a new coverslip.

Bibliography

Carson FL. Nuclear and xytoplasmic staining. In: Carson FL. *Histotechnology: A Self-Instructional Text.* 2nd ed. Chicago, IL: American Society of Clinical Pathologists; 1997.

Dapson R. Troubleshooting Problems in Processing and Staining [workshop handout]. Columbus, MD: National Society for Histotechnology; 1997.

Feldman A. H&E stain. In: *NSH-CAP HQIP: A Final Critique.* Northfield, IL: College of American Pathologists; 2004:20-25.

Guidelines for Hematoxylin and Eosin Staining [instruction booklet]. Columbus, MD: National Society for Histotechnology; 1994.

Sheehan DC, Hrapchak BB. Nuclear and cytoplasmic stains. In: Sheehan DC, Hrapchak BB, eds. *Theory and Practice of Histotechnology.* 2nd ed. Columbus, OH: Battelle Press; 1980.

Vesey J. Back to the Basics: Troubleshooting the H&E Stain [teleconference presentation and handout]. San Antonio, TX: University of Texas Health Science Center at San Antonio; 2004.

Wilson I, Gamble M. The hematoxylins and eosin. In: Bancroft JD, Gamble M, eds. *Theory and Practice of Histological Techniques.* 5th ed. New York, NY: Churchill Livingstone; 2002.

ACKNOWLEDGEMENTS:
Thank you to Ada Feldman for the NSH/CAP HistoQIP Final Critique (see Bibliography). Some information for this chapter is taken directly from that critique, as are some images and illustrations. I also thank Robert Lott for providing images and content.

Gram Stain

Robert L. Lott

Bacteria are single-celled microorganisms found in soil, air, food, and in all animals and humans. They are often difficult in discern microscopically in infected tissues, staining a light blue-gray with the hematoxylin and eosin (H&E) stain (Figure 5.1). The most common tissue response to infection in humans is acute inflammation with neutrophils. The H&E stain will reveal this inflammatory response, as well as other changes, such as necrosis, abscess, granulomas, or an increase in macrophages or lymphocytes. Other types of microorganisms, such as fungi, viruses, and parasites, can also cause these pathological reactions. Because most bacteria are small (average size range is 0.2 to 10 μm in length and 1 to 2 μm in diameter), viewing them with a light microscope can be difficult, often requiring special stains and/or high magnification.[1-3]

Various stains can be used to visualize and possibly differentiate bacteria. Carbolfuchsin stains, such as Ziehl-Neelsen and Kinyoun, will distinguish the acid-fast bacteria. Silver impregnation methods, such as Steiner or Warthin-Starry, stain all bacteria black. They are particularly useful in screening for the presence of small numbers of bacteria and are essential for staining spirochetes. Giemsa and Diff-Quik® will nondifferentially stain all bacteria blue. Immunohistochemical stains will provide a high degree of specificity and sensitivity in the detection and identification of bacteria. However, the Gram stain is a fast simple method that not only colors the bacteria for visualization but also separates them into two color groups based on cell wall characteristics. The Gram stain is usually the first test performed for bacterial identification. Gram stains can be performed in minutes, whereas culture results and definitive identification may take several days.

Hans Christian Gram, a bacteriologist from Denmark, developed and published his work on the stain in 1884. The Gram stain has become an important tool in bacterial taxonomy, distinguishing between gram-positive bacteria, which remain colored after the staining procedure, and gram-negative bacteria, which do not retain the dye. The differential staining reflects the composition of the cell wall that surrounds the bacterium and gives it strength (Figure 5-2). Recent studies have revealed that the cell wall of gram-negative bacteria is composed of a thin layer of pep-

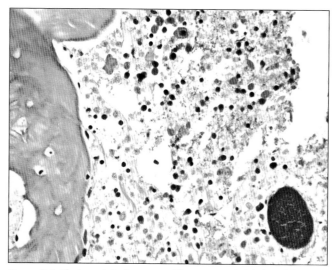

Figure 5.1. The bacteria in this section of bone appear slightly basophilic, staining a light blue-gray with the H&E stain.

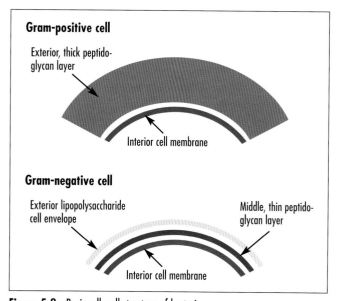

Figure 5.2. Basic cell wall structure of bacteria.

tidoglycan sandwiched between an "outer" lipopolysaccharide cell envelope and the inner cell membrane. The gram-positive cell wall is thicker, composed of multiple interlinked layers of peptidoglycan; however, it lacks the outer lipopolysaccharide cell envelope.[4]

Peptidoglycan, also known as *murein,* is a polymer consisting of sugars and amino acids. It serves a structural role, much like a chain-link fence, in the bacterial cell wall, giving it shape and structural strength, as well as resisting the osmotic pressure of the cytoplasm. Both gram-negative and gram-positive bacteria have a peptidoglycan layer; however, the arrangement of this layer in the cell wall differs. In gram-positive bacteria, the peptidoglycan is a heavily cross-linked woven structure that encases the cell in many layers. It is relatively thick, with the peptidoglycan accounting for 50% of the weight of the cell and 90% of the weight of the cell wall. Electron micrographs show the peptidoglycan to be 20 to 80 nm thick. In gram-negative bacteria, the peptidoglycan is thinner, accounting for only 15% to 20% of the cell wall, and it is only intermittently cross-linked. However, in both cases, peptidoglycan is not a barrier to solutes or dyes because the openings in the polymer are large enough for most molecules to pass through.[5]

In the Gram stain procedure, crystal violet, which is the purple, positively charged dye, binds to the negatively charged phospholipids, lipoproteins, and proteins found in all cell walls and becomes trapped in the layers of peptidoglycan found in both types of bacteria. Iodine, subsequently added as a mordant, complexes with the crystal violet, forming a large, water-insoluble precipitate (CV-I_3 complex). The large size of this CV-I_3 complex makes it difficult to remove. This step is commonly referred to as "fixing" the dye. However, subsequent treatment with a decolorizer, an organic solvent of ethanol, acetone, ether, or a mixture of these, dissolves the outer lipid layer from gram-negative cells. The removal of the lipid layer enhances the leaching of the CV-I_3 complex from the thin peptidoglycan layer into the surrounding organic solvent. In contrast, the solvent dehydrates the much thicker gram-positive cell walls, closing off the pores as the cell wall shrinks during dehydration. As a result, the diffusion of the large CV-I_3 complex is blocked, and the gram-positive bacteria remain stained.[6] In addition, polymers of acids in the cell walls of gram-positive bacteria increase the binding of the positively charged dyes. The thickness of the peptidoglycan layers and the presence or absence of the outer lipid envelope are the key factors in Gram staining.

From the above description, it is clear that the decolorization step is the one most likely to cause problems in the Gram stain. The timing of this step is critical. Generally, decolorization of tissue sections should not exceed 5 seconds, or 3 to 4 quick dips. Prolonged exposure to the solvent used in this step will remove all the stain from both types of bacteria. Some gram-positive species have the tendency to lose the stain more easily than others and can appear as a mixture of gram-positive and gram-negative bacteria. These bacteria are often termed *gram-variable.* Insufficient decolorization can,

however, make gram-negative organisms appear falsely gram-positive. Other problems specifically related to the decolorization step include a low concentration of crystal violet, making gram-positive organisms more susceptible to over-decolorization. Insufficient exposure to iodine and/or lack of available iodine in solution can prevent crystal violet from complexing or bonding firmly within the cell wall, thus making gram-positive organisms more susceptible to decolorization. The iodine solution should always be stored tightly capped. To ensure reliable Gram stain results, fresh iodine should be used.[7]

Finally, a counterstain of basic fuchsin is applied to give decolorized gram-negative bacteria a pink-red color. Some laboratories use safranin or neutral red as a counterstain instead. Basic fuchsin stains many gram-negative bacteria more intensely than does safranin, making them easier to see. Bacteria that are poorly stained by safranin, such as *Haemophilus* species, *Legionella* species, and some anaerobic bacteria, are readily stained by basic fuchsin but not by safranin. Insufficient counterstaining can fail to stain gram negative bacteria and background material, whereas excessive counterstaining will leach the CV-I_3 complex from gram-positive bacteria and stain them with safranin, thus making them falsely appear gram-negative. Generally, counterstaining should not exceed 1 to 2 minutes. Prolonged washing between any of these steps can cause over-decolorization.

The traditional Gram stain works very well on fresh smears of exudate material or on imprints from tissue. In contrast, this stain is more difficult to perform properly on tissue sections because of the fixation and processing through dehydrants and clearants to paraffin. Processing tends to alter the outer membranes of the bacteria present in tissue sections. As a result, variations of the traditional Gram stain have been developed to compensate for these alterations. The most common are the Brown-Hopps (B&H) and Brown and Brenn (B&B) procedures.[3] Gram-negative bacteria are demonstrated better with the B&H staining method, whereas the B&B method is often preferred for gram-positive organisms.[3] In practice, it may be best to use both stains to detect bacteria in tissue sections. Other techniques devised for tissue, such as the Gram-Twort[8] technique, yield good color contrast of gram-negative bacteria against the tissue background but are time consuming, and over- or under-differentiation can occur. The MacCallum-Goodpasture[9] procedure produces good results but has lost popularity because of its requirement for several dangerous chemicals, such as aniline (a potential carcinogen), phenol, 40% formaldehyde, and saturated aqueous picric acid solution. Lillie's[10] "Gram Stain for Sections" uses a unique crystal violet-ammonium oxalate solution and Weigert's iodine, rather than Gram's iodine. The gram-positive organisms stain very intensely. The safranin or neutral-red counterstain is not as intense as basic fuchsin, which makes identification of gram-negative bacteria easier. With any variation devised for paraffin sections, considerable experience and practice is needed for accurate differentiation and to achieve optimal results.

All methods have the drawback that under- or over-differentiation can occur in the acetone-alcohol used after the CV-I₃ treatment. However, one of the most common mistakes with Gram stains performed on tissue sections is to allow completed, well-stained slides to be overdehydrated before clearing and coverslipping. The alcohols will continue to decolorize the CV-I₃ complex from gram-positive bacteria and remove counterstain from gram-negative bacteria. Slides must be passed quickly through these dehydrating steps. Experienced technologists will blot the water from each section and use only a few quick dips in absolute alcohol before moving to xylene and then coverslipping. The short dips in alcohol or even acetone at the end of the procedure should not be skipped, however, because they aid in removing excess red dye from the background, so that gram-negative bacteria may be more easily recognized. Once the section is in xylene, the decolorization will stop unless the xylene is contaminated with alcohol.

In general, gram-positive bacteria (blue) are easier to see against the predominantly red-and-yellow background of tissue and inflammation than are gram-negative bacteria (red), especially if the gram-negative bacteria stain poorly. Certain bacterial pathogens are notorious for staining poorly with the usual gram-negative counterstains, for example, *Legionella*, *Bordetella*, *Bacteroides*, and *Brucella*.[3] Engbaek et al compared Gram stain techniques for suitability of use with paraffin sections, with emphasis on the adequacy of staining of the problematic gram-negative organisms; they recommended a modification of the B&H method.[11] Chandler suggests that the depth and intensity of staining of weakly gram-negative organisms can be improved by increasing the concentration of the basic fuchsin solution 10-fold (from 0.1% to 1.0%).[12]

Pathologists often use tissue Gram stains as a simple screening tool for the presence of bacteria rather than as an attempt to truly characterize and classify the organisms (Table 5.1). Interpretation of tissue Gram stains presents a unique set of problems, and caution must be used. Bacteria found in areas of extensive necrosis may be dead or dying, which causes damage to their cell walls and, as a result, they will stain variably. Organisms that have been treated with antibiotics may stain in an equally unpredictable manner. Assuming proper control material is used, bacteria found in tissue sections that retain the CV-I₃ complex and stain blue-black can safely be characterized as gram-positive. However, it is often impossible to tell whether red-stained organisms are truly gram-negative or represent dead and dying gram-positive bacteria.

Table 5.1. Classification of Some Important Bacterial Genera[13]

| Gram-positive | | Gram-negative | | |
Cocci	Bacilli	Cocci	Bacilli	Coccobacilli
Staphylococcus	Bacillus	Neisseria	Escherichia	Brucella
Streptococcus	Clostridium		Klebsiella	Bordetella
Enterococcus	Corynebacterium		Salmonella	Haemophilus
	Mycobacterium		Shigella	
	Lactobacillus		Proteus	
	Listeria		Pseudomonas	
			Vibrio	
			Pasturella	
			Campylobacter	

The Gram stain and its variations work on the following principle:

Step 1: A **crystal violet** solution is applied to the tissue, staining all cells and tissue structures blue. This cationic, positively charged dye binds to the negatively charged phospholipids, lipoproteins, proteins, and peptidoglycans found in all cell walls, including all bacteria.

Step 2: Next, an aqueous **iodine** solution, composed of iodine and potassium iodide, is applied. The tri-iodine ion (I₃⁻) binds with the crystal violet dye, creating a water-insoluble crystal violet–iodine (CV-I₃) complex. At this point, all the cells are stained blue-black.

Step 3: After careful blotting of excess water, **differentiation (or decolorization) in an organic solvent,** such as ethanol, acetone, ether, or cellosolve, is used to extract the CV-I₃ complex. Gram-positive bacteria, with their thick cell wall layers of lipoproteins and peptidoglycans, resist this extraction longer than do gram-negative bacteria. All other eukaryotic cells and cell components lose the CV-I₃ complex during the organic solvent differentiation.

Step 4: Next, a **red dye,** such as basic fuchsin, safranin O, neutral red, new fuchsin, or pararosanilin, is applied. Variations of the Gram stain method for tissue sections use different counterstains to achieve staining of gram-negative bacteria, which will be stained pink to red, as will cell cytoplasm and fibrin. The **excess red color of background cells can be removed or lightened** by briefly dipping the slides in an organic solvent such as acetone, alcohol, or cellosolve. Care must be taken to keep the time short, because extended time in the organic solvent can remove the red color from gram-negative bacteria. The B&H procedure uses a **Gallego solution—** a formalin, glacial acetic acid, and water solution—to

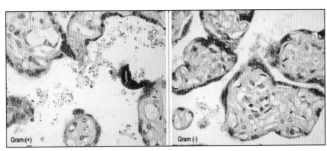

Figure 5.3. Homemade Gram stain control sections using placenta are well stained with Lillie's method. Blue-black gram-positive *Streptococcus* (cocci) are on the left and red gram-negative *E coli* (bacilli) are on the right. Cell nuclei appear red.

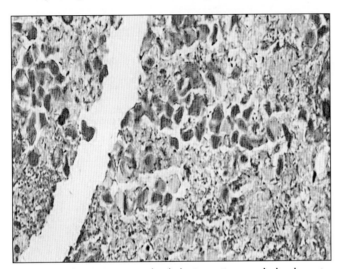

Figure 5.4. This section is stained with the Brown-Hopps method and contains many gram-negative *Pseudomonas aeruginosa*. Note that the rods appear more violet than red with this technique. Cell nuclei appear red.

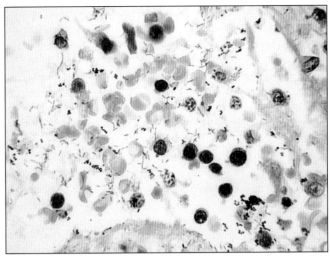

Figure 5.5. This section of lung is stained with the Brown and Brenn method. Gram-positive cocci, present in clusters, appear blue-black. Gram-negative rods are a distinct pink-red. Both contrast well against the delicate yellow background. Cell nuclei appear red.

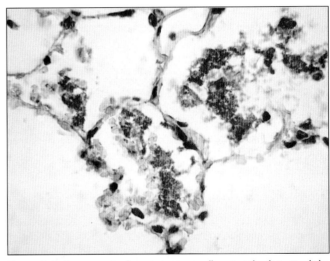

Figure 5.6. Gram-negative bacteria contrast well against the distinctive light-green background in this section of lung, which is stained with the Gram-Twort method. Cell nuclei appear red.

"fix" the red dye in the gram-negative bacteria and to remove some of the red color from the background, which also has the effect of changing the red color of the gram-negative bacteria to a reddish-violet color.

An additional or optional **yellow counterstain,** such as picric acid or tartrazine can be used on tissue sections to stain the background yellow. This stain often increases the contrast between the red-stained gram-negative bacteria and the background.

Controls

Ideally, control material should contain both gram-positive and gram-negative bacteria, each with unique and "opposite" morphological criteria. Known gram-positive cocci paired with known gram-negative rods, or the reverse, is ideal. There are several methods available for producing "homemade" Gram stain controls that result in separate, side-by-side tissue sections containing morphologically opposite control material. Alternately, tissue blocks that contain known gram-positive or gram-negative species can be combined and sectioned together to serve as adequate control material. It should be regarded as an act of negligence to send out a Gram-stained section without a proper control.[14]

What Should Be Seen in a Good Gram Stain

The differentiation of bacteria into either the gram-positive or the gram-negative group is fundamental to identification. Unfortunately, the Gram stain methodology, although simple to perform, is prone to error. The operator-dependent nature of this procedure can be addressed by attention to detail and the use of controls

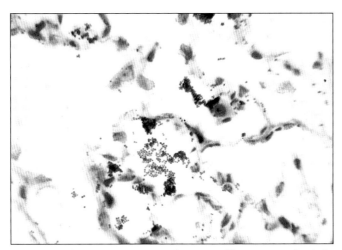

Figure 5.7. The gram-positive cocci in this section of lung are stained with the Brown and Brenn method but have been over-decolorized, making them appear gram-negative.

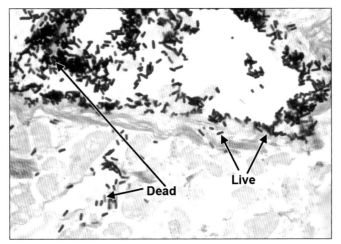

Figure 5.8. Gram-positive *Clostridium perfringens* is stained with the Brown and Brenn method. Occasional red-stained bacteria are seen, but these are probably dead and have lost their Gram positivity. The blue-black color of the live rods is demonstrated very well.

with the test. Optimization of the chosen Gram stain variation is essential to performing this technique well when using paraffin sections. Only by making, using, or combining blocks with known gram-positive and gram-negative organisms can any method be optimized. Sections should demonstrate distinctively stained blue-black gram-positive bacteria. Sections should also demonstrate well-defined, red-stained gram-negative bacteria that can be uniquely identified or contrasted against a similarly stained tissue background. Ideally, different bacterial strains will be shown in different colors, affording the arbitrary division into two main groups and aiding their identification. Good Gram stains by various techniques are demonstrated in Figures 5.3 through 5.6.

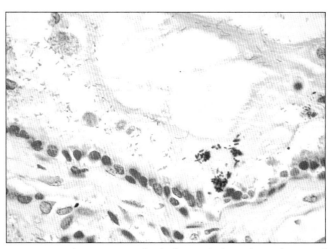

Figure 5.9. In this section, stained with Lillie's method, it is obvious that most of the once gram-positive rods are dead and are stained red with the counterstain. The few remaining live gram-positive bacteria are distinctly blue-black. This appearance is very common in tissue Gram stains.

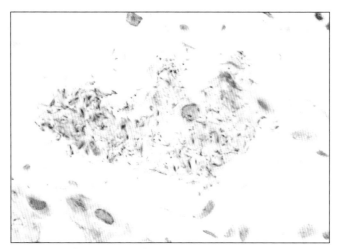

Figure 5.10. This section, stained with the Brown-Hopps method, was allowed to sit in the alcohol series before clearing and coverslipping. As a result, staining of the gram-positive organisms has been partially damaged, with some bacteria completely decolorized. Cell nuclei have lost the expected red color.

Problems Encountered With the Gram Stain

PROBLEM: No Gram-Positive Bacteria are Staining in Known Gram-Positive Control Slide or in Patient's Tissue Specimen

APPEARANCE: The known gram-positive bacteria are not properly stained blue-black or are stained red with the counterstain (Figures 5.7 through 5.10).

CAUSES:

- The tissue section was over-decolorized in Step 3 with the organic solvent.

- The bacteria are dead, old, or being treated with antibiotics. Because of the treatment, the cell walls of the bacteria have been compromised and cannot resist decolorization.

- There was an error in the iodine solution step.
- Completed stains were allowed to sit or were dehydrated too long in the alcohol series before clearing and coverslipping.

SOLUTIONS:

- Reduce the time in organic solvent. Wash slide quickly and thoroughly with fresh water. Use a slightly "slower" organic solvent, such as an acetone-alcohol mixture, or alcohol instead of acetone, or acetone diluted with water. This solvent substitution will add a degree of control to the decolorization step.
- For dead or dying bacteria, increase the time in the crystal violet and iodine solutions, reduce the time in the decolorizer, or use a diluted decolorizer.
- Ensure that the iodine solution is made correctly and properly applied. Seal after use. Iodine solutions lose their efficacy rapidly when exposed to air. Use a freshly made or newly purchased iodine solution.
- When finishing the stain, after completion of Step 4, quickly dehydrate slides through alcohol to xylene. This process may need to be done one slide at a time to effectively prevent over-decolorization of gram-positive organisms.

COMMENTS: Gram-positive staining (Steps 1 and 2) is the easiest portion of the protocol to perform correctly; however, it can be undone completely by over-decolorization. Decolorization is the most operator-dependent step of the process and the one that is most likely to be performed incorrectly. If the patient is on antibiotic treatment, the drugs will attack the cell wall of the bacteria, causing it to lose its ability to retain the black CV-I_3 complex. Gram-positive bacteria may no longer stain blue-black and will pick up the red color of the counterstain. Dead and dying gram-positive bacteria will often not retain the CV-I_3 complex and appear gram-negative. If an organic solvent, like alcohol and acetone, is used for the original decolorization of the CV-I_3 complex, it is logical to assume that when slides are allowed to sit in alcohol before clearing and coverslipping, gram-positive organisms will be further, or perhaps completely, decolorized. Always use a control slide with "viable" gram-positive and gram-negative bacteria so that the result may be assessed.

PROBLEM: Background Structures Retaining a Blue-Black Color

APPEARANCE: The background of the tissue section is not completely decolorized by the organic solvent (Step 3), and therefore there is no contrast between the distinct blue-black color of the gram-positive bacteria and the background. Nuclei, which should be the color of the

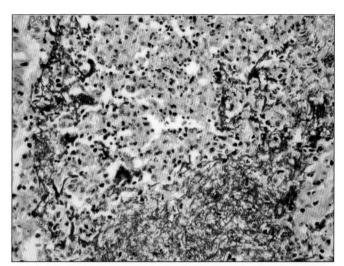

Figure 5.11. This Gram-stained section shows the effects of failing to decolorize with acetone to remove the CV-I_3 complex, resulting in poor staining. A blue web of the complex is still present along with a purple haze in the background. Note that most cell nuclei are still darkened with the complex rather than being the expected red color.

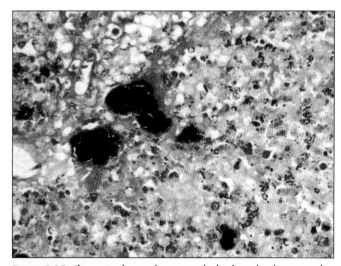

Figure 5.12. This section has not been properly decolorized with acetone-alcohol. Large aggregates of the CV-I_3 complex remain against a dark purple background that could not be stained with the red counterstain. Cell nuclei are dark, having retained the complex as well.

counterstain (red), retain the dark blue-black color of the CV-I_3 complex (Figures 5.11 and 5.12).

CAUSES:

- Under-decolorization occurred with the organic solvent (acetone or alcohol).
- The crystal violet dried on the slide, creating an insoluble end product.

SOLUTIONS:

- Increase the time in the decolorizing solution, or use a faster organic solvent. Use an undiluted organic solvent, such as acetone.

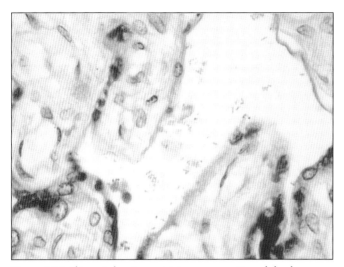

Figure 5.13. This control section containing gram-negative rods has been over-decolorized by allowing it to sit in the alcohols before clearing and coverslipping. The nuclei and background have lost most of their expected coloring. (Compare with Figure 5.3.)

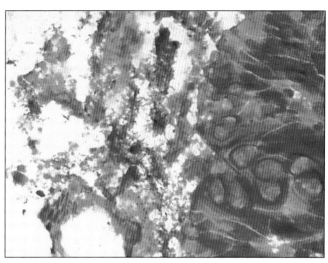

Figure 5.14. The counterstain in this section stained with the Brown and Brenn method has not been properly decolorized. The residual red dye causes a lack of contrast between the gram-negative bacteria and the background. (Compare with Figure 5.15.)

- Do not allow the stains to dry on the slides during or between steps.

COMMENTS: Denser tissue components, such as keratin, often retain a portion of the blue-black color and can cause reduced contrast. However, dye retention is usually caused by drying of the section between the crystal violet step and the iodine step or before the decolorization step. Many procedures recommend that the slide be blotted before decolorization. Blotting should be performed with a damp paper or sponge. Care must be taken that drying does not occur at this point.

PROBLEM: Gram-Negative Bacteria Not Staining or Difficult to See Against Background

APPEARANCE: Known gram-negative bacteria are not stained red, or the red dye solution has stained tissue elements and structures in the background the same color. There is lack of contrast between the red bacteria and the background, making the bacteria difficult to identify (Figures 5.13 and 5.14).

CAUSES:

- Sections have been kept too long in the dehydrant after the red dye (Step 4).
- The CV-I₃ complex was not completely removed (Step 3) from gram-negative bacteria, so the red dye cannot stain it (see "Problem" above).
- There was inadequate exposure to dehydrant or Gallego solution.
- Counterstain, such as picric acid or tartrazine, was not used to provide contrast.
- There was an error with the red dye.

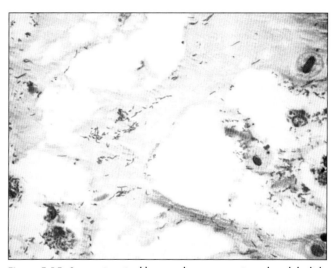

Figure 5.15. Contrast is optimal between the gram-negative rods and the light yellow background in this Gram stain performed with the Brown and Brenn method.

SOLUTIONS:

- Reduce time in all of the dehydrants used after the red dye step. Dehydrants will decolorize the red dye staining of gram-negative organisms, just as they will decolorize the blue-black CV-I₃ complex of the gram-positive organisms (see above).
- Use Gallego solution to set the red dye in gram-negative bacteria, making it more resistant to decolorization by the dehydrant. Gallego solution will also slightly leech the red dye from background.
- Increase time in organic solvent to efficiently remove the CV-I₃ complex.

- Quickly decolorize counterstain, using quick dips in 2 or 3 alcohol containers.

- Increase time in red dye, or prepare fresh red dye solution to ensure concentration is adequate.

- Always use a control slide that contains both gram-positive and gram-negative bacteria so that the end result may be assessed. Use of the B&H modification turns gram-negative bacteria slightly violet in color and may improve contrast with background structures.

COMMENTS: Alcohols or dehydrants used to finish the procedure can damage gram-positive organisms; however, it is the staining of gram-negative bacteria that is affected most. The finishing steps must be performed quickly or the delicate pink-red gram-negative bacteria will be decolorized. Sections that have been overexposed to dehydrants at the end of the procedure will also show diminished red staining of cell nuclei. This problem is one of the most common errors in the Gram staining of tissue samples.

References

1. Carson FL. *Histotechnology: A Self-Instructional Text.* 2nd ed. Chicago, IL: American Society of Clinical Pathologists; 1997: 180-189.

2. Sheehan DC, Hrapchak BB. *Theory and Practice of Histotechnology.* 2nd ed. Columbus, OH: Battelle Press; 1980: 233-235.

3. Winn WD. Current concepts in pathologic diagnosis: bacterial diseases. *J Histotechnol.* 1995;18:241-246.

4. Beveridge TJ. Structure of bacterial surfaces and how it influences their Gram stainability. Presented at National Society for Histotechnology Symposium; September 23, 2001; Charlotte, NC.

5. Beveridge TJ, Graham LL. Surface layers of bacteria. *Microbiol Rev.* 1991;55(4):684-705.

6. Davies JA, Anderson GK, Beveridge TJ, Clark HC. Chemical mechanism of the Gram stain and synthesis of a new electron-opaque marker for electron microscopy which replaces the iodine mordant of the stain. *J Bacteriol.* 1983;156(2):837-845.

7. McClelland R. Gram's stain: the key to microbiology. *MLO Med Lab Obs.* 2001;183(7):20-22, 25-28; quiz 30-31.

8. Twort FW. An improved neutral red, light green doublestain for staining animal parasites, microorganisms and tissue. *J State Medicine.* 1924;32:351.

9. MacCallum WG. MacCallum-Goodpasture method for Gram positive and Gram negative bacteria. *JAMA.* 1919;72:193.

10. Lillie RD. *Histopathologic Technic and Practical Histochemistry.* 3rd ed. New York, NY: McGraw-Hill; 1965: 566-569.

11. Engbaek K, Johansen KS, Jensen ME. A new technique for Gram staining paraffin-embedded tissue. *J Clin Pathol.* 1979;32:187-190.

12. Chandler FW. Infectious disease pathology: morphologic and molecular approaches to diagnosis. *J Histotechnol.* 1995;18(3):183-186.

13. Bancroft JD, Gamble M. *Theory and Practice of Histological Techniques.* 5th ed. New York, NY: Churchill Livingstone; 2002: 325-329.

14. Bancroft J, Stevens A. *Theory and Practice of Histologic Techniques.* 2nd ed. New York, NY: Churchill Livingstone; 1982: 280-283.

ACKNOWLEDGEMENT:
A special thank you to Peggy A. Wenk, HTL(ASCP)SLS, who wrote the original article on Gram stains for the 2005-B NSH/CAP HistoQIP Final Critique. Although modified, some of the introductory material for this chapter is taken directly from that article, as are several of the images.

Mycobacteria

Robert L. Lott

The rise in the number of mycobacterial infections in recent years has increased the need for reliable and reproducible methods for the demonstration of these bacteria. The resurgence in mycobacterial infections is due to a number of factors, including homelessness, drug use, immunodeficiency disorders, and mobility of individuals from countries where there is a high number of tubercular cases. Generally, it is the atypical mycobacteria that infect immunocompromised individuals. With the acquired immune deficiency syndrome (AIDS) epidemic, atypical mycobacteria have taken on new importance with the recognition that the *Mycobacterium avium-intracellulare* complex (MAC) results in the most common AIDS-associated systemic bacterial infection. Atypical mycobacteria can cause tuberculosis-like or leprosy-like diseases and often are not susceptible to certain common antituberculous antibiotics.

Histologically, in a MAC infection, one often sees non-granulomatous lesions with numerous organisms. MAC infection is characterized by preferential involvement of the organs of the mononuclear phagocyte system, including lymph nodes, spleen, liver, and bone marrow.[1] *M tuberculosis* infects the lung, is distributed systemically within macrophages, and survives intracellularly. Cell-mediated immunity develops, which causes the development of granulomas or "tubercles" (Figure 6.1). In culture, *M tuberculosis* grows very slowly, producing distinct nonpigmented colonies only after several weeks. It can be differentiated from most other mycobacteria by the production of niacin. A rapid alternative to culture is gene amplification by polymerase chain reaction. *M tuberculosis* can cause disease in immunocompetent individuals and is transmitted person-to-person in airborne droplets.

Mycobacteria are rod-shaped bacilli that can also form filaments. Depending on the species, the microscopic appearance may be long, slender, straight, curved, or even granular. The structure of the cell wall of these bacilli is unique and important because it is largely responsible for the staining reaction. Long-chained fatty acids called mycolic acids are present in these walls, along with a peptidoglycan layer. This lipoid capsule is of such high molecular weight that it is "waxy" at room temperature, rendering the cell walls hydrophobic.

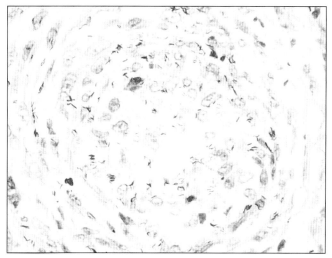

Figure 6.1. A good stain for *M tuberculosis,* using the Ziehl-Neelsen technique, is illustrated in this figure. The organisms are distinctly red against a clear background. The methylene blue counterstain only stains the nuclei of the cells in the background.

Logically then, penetration of the dye into the cell can be enhanced by heat treatment or by incorporation of a detergent into the dye solution, which reduces surface tension and increases porosity. This waxy coat also influences stain removal. Carbolfuchsin is more soluble in the lipids of the cell wall than in acid-alcohol, therefore it is readily removed from other bacteria that lack the waxy capsule.[2] The *Mycobacterium* species retain the stain when using acid and/or alcohol, and thus they are referred to as *acid-fast* bacteria. The lipid content also makes these organisms very resistant to destruction by drying, chemicals, and antimicrobial drugs.

The best known and most widely used method for demonstrating acid-fast bacteria is the Ziehl-Neelsen technique. It incorporates heating of a carbolfuchsin solution, literally forcing it into the waxy cell wall. Although it is clear that the original authors of this method intended that the stain solution be heated, extended or prolonged exposure works as well.[2] However, both Fite and Lillie[3] have observed that heated, or previously heated and cooled, carbolfuchsin solutions stain more brilliantly than unheated ones. This observation suggests that "supersaturation" may play an important role in brilliancy of staining.[3] No heating of the carbolfuchsin is required with the Kinyoun technique; often referred to as the "cold" Ziehl-Neelsen, it uses an increased concentration (approximately four-fold) of dye in the carbolfuchsin instead of heating.[4] Both methods call for the application of a phenyl methane dye (new fuchsin, rosaniline, or pararosanaline) in a phenol solution. Concerns over the use of the toxic solvent phenol in the laboratory have led several investigators to advocate its substitution with liquid detergents or surfactants.[5,6] The use of either phenol or detergent will reduce surface tension and aid dye penetration into the waxy, hard-to-stain, acid-fast bacilli as well as into all other tissue structures. Decolorization by an acid-alcohol solution, usually 0.5% to 1.0% HCl in 70% alcohol, follows the application of the dye complex and thorough washing. During decolorization, all tissue structures, except those that are acid-fast, are rendered colorless. Red blood cells are especially resistant to complete decolorization by acid-alcohol and appear reddish-orange. The concentration of acid and the length of time in the decolorizing solution can lead to variable staining. Properly stained organisms will resist over-decolorization with acid-alcohol, but "partially" acid-fast organisms can be completely decolorized with minimal treatment. The final step is the application of a counterstain (methylene blue, malachite green, light green, or fast green FCF) for contrast.

Other microorganisms and other cellular structures and materials may also be demonstrated with acid-fast techniques. These include *Cryptosporidium*, *Nocardia* species, lipofuscin (ceroid), intranuclear inclusion bodies in cases of chronic lead poisoning, and Russell bodies present in plasma cells.

The leprosy bacillus, *M leprae*, along with other microorganisms like *Nocardia* and *Cryptosporidium*, are much less acid- and alcohol-fast than other mycobacteria. They are commonly referred to as "partially" acid-fast and are completely decolorized by the standard Ziehl-Neelsen technique; therefore, a "modified" Ziehl-Neelsen is necessary for their demonstration. The Fite technique, or one of its modifications,[7] is recommended for the demonstration of these microbes. Mineral oil or vegetable oil is used in the deparaffinization of slides and appears to provide a protective coating around these organisms. This modification helps avoid over-decolorization of organisms but can cause staining artifacts if the oil is not effectively blotted and washed before exposure to carbolfuchsin. Decolorization of the background is accomplished by use of an aqueous sulfuric acid solution that allows for better control during differentiation.[8] Alcohol should not be used during hydration or dehydration of the sections. In addition, it is important to avoid over-counterstaining with methylene blue because removal with alcohol is precluded. The Fite stain is preferred in the clinical laboratory for partially acid-fast bacteria because the often-referenced Putt stain may produce false-positive results.[4]

A real concern with the detection of mycobacteria in tissue sections is that they are usually present only in small numbers, and considerable time must be spent scanning the section. The fluorescent techniques of Kuper and May[9] or Truant et al[10] are popular because the bright, orange-yellow fluorescent organisms stand out clearly against a dark background and can be visualized quite well with a fluorescence microscope at 20x or 40x magnification. Screening of large expanses of tissue is, therefore, facilitated by use of the fluorochrome dyes auramine and rhodamine. Staining depends on exactly the same mechanisms as those of the carbolfuchsin stains. Several authors have called the auramine-rhodamine method "exquisitely sensitive" because it can demonstrate a single "red-snapper" in sections that would normally be considered negative for the presence of acid-fast organisms.[11] Having worked extensively with fluorochrome detection methods for mycobacteria while developing microwave modifications, Churukian observed that the fluorochrome methods are more likely to stain dead and dying organisms than are the carbolfuchsin methods.[12] He also found that rhodamine B, unless present in only very small amounts in the staining solution, can actually act to quench fluorescence of the organisms.[12] Apart from the inherent problems with fluorescence microscopy, where some expertise is necessary, it seems odd that what many regard as the most sensitive method for demonstrating mycobacteria in tissue sections may be utilized the least.

Are these conventional histologic staining methods an adequate tool for detection of mycobacteria in tissue sections? Most pathologists doubt the true sensitivity when using them, especially when the number of bacilli is low. One study compared detection of mycobacteria in tissue sections of 30 patients with tuberculosis lesions using reverse transcriptase-polymerase chain reaction (positive in 83% of cases) versus Ziehl-Neelsen staining (positive in 40% of cases).[13] Some researchers have suspected that the organic solvents used in processing might affect the stainability of mycobacteria, which seems reasonable because the target of the acid-fast dyes (carbolfuchsin, auramine, or rhodamine) is the mycolic acid-lipid envelope on the bacterial surface.[6] This mycolate is soluble in organic agents[14] and might be more or less extracted from the cell wall. Moreover, reports seem to indicate that the Fite method, the alternative technique that uses less alcohol and xylene in the staining and mounting process, has a higher sensitivity than Ziehl-Neelsen staining.[15,16]

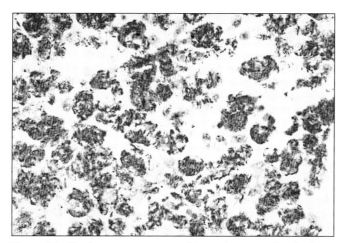

Figure 6.2. *Mycobacterium avium-intracellulare* is demonstrated in this figure with the Ziehl-Neelsen method. Infection with this organism is generally associated with acquired immune deficiency syndrome (AIDS). Infections with the *M avium-intracellulare* complex are less likely to produce visible granulomas, and the lesions often consist of clusters of macrophages filled with numerous mycobacteria.

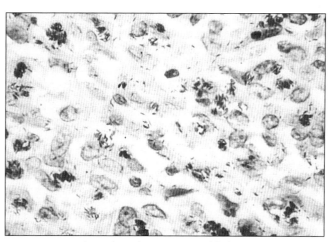

Figure 6.3. A good stain for *M leprae* using a modified Fite technique is shown in this figure. These partially acid-fast organisms are well demonstrated; the nuclei in the background are lightly stained with Mayer hematoxylin.

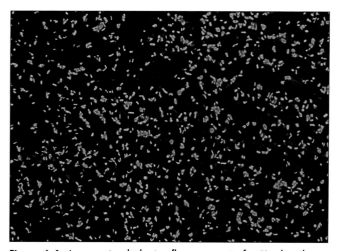

Figure 6.4. An auramine-rhodamine fluorescent stain for *M tuberculosis* is shown in this figure. The organisms are demonstrated as bright yellow rods against a dark background. A skilled microscopist, using strict morphologic criteria, is necessary to adequately evaluate this stain.

In 2002, Fukunaga et al demonstrated quantitatively that both formalin fixation and xylene processing markedly reduced the sensitivity of acid-fast staining, regardless of the method used (carbolfuchsin or fluorescence).[13] This finding suggests that the number of mycobacteria in tissue sections may be significantly underestimated with conventional acid-fast staining techniques.

Controls

When searching for any of these microorganisms—the atypical or the partially acid-fast mycobacteria—it is advisable to use the standard Ziehl-Neelsen method or the Fite method (or one of its modifications) and a fluorescent method to increase the chances of detection.[4] With any of these techniques, it is important to use a positive and a negative control slide. The best control slide should include a tissue known to be positive (tissue specific) for the organism to be stained, with a moderate number of organisms, in combination with a negative tissue control slide (eg, tonsil or uterus). A negative tissue control slide is important because tap water, water baths, and the reagents may contain "wayward" acid-fast bacilli. Portions of the slide apart from the tissue section should be observed in order to identify such contaminants.

What Should Be Seen in a Good Stain for Mycobacteria

The acid-fast organisms should stain bright red with the Ziehl-Neelsen, Kinyoun, and Fite methods, while all other structures are colored according to the counter-stain used. The most common counterstain is methylene blue, and, when used, it should color only the nuclei. The background connective tissue and stroma should be clear or colorless to provide the best contrast in a well-stained section. The fluorochrome methods yield a bright yellow or orange-red organism on a dark black background. Caution should always be used when interpreting stains for acid-fast bacilli (AFB). The reviewer should always use recognized morphologic criteria for the identification of the microorganisms. Good mycobacterial stains by the various techniques are demonstrated in Figures 6.1 through 6.4.

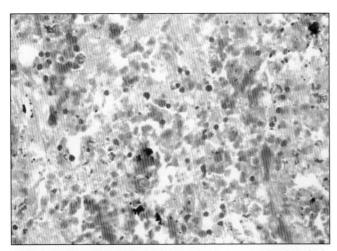

Figure 6.5. The acid-fast bacilli in this section do not contrast well with the background because the tissue is poorly decolorized and the counterstain is too light in this Ziehl-Neelsen stain.

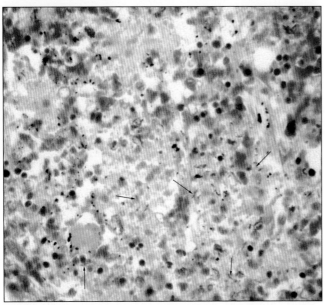

Figure 6.6. The acid-fast bacilli present in this section of lung (arrows) are inconspicuous because of the presence of pigment and incompletely decolorized red blood cells in the background.

Problems Encountered With Stains for Mycobacteria

PROBLEM: Incomplete Decolorization

APPEARANCE: Background tissue structures have not been completely decolorized, making organisms difficult to visualize or masking them completely (Figures 6.5 and 6.6).

CAUSE:

• Sections did not spend adequate time in acid-alcohol solution.

SOLUTIONS:

• Increase time in acid-alcohol solution or use a stronger solution.

• Wash sections thoroughly in warm water both before and after decolorization.

COMMENTS: Most procedures recommend a 1% or 0.5% acid-alcohol solution for decolorization. Make sure that sections are exposed to the solution for adequate time to render a basically colorless background so that acid-fast organisms may be visualized. Check microscopically before proceeding. Even in a well-stained section, red blood cells usually retain a bit of red color and may pose a background problem.

PROBLEM: Over-Decolorization

APPEARANCE: The organisms in known acid-fast control sections are only lightly stained or not stained at all (Figure 6.7).

CAUSES:

• Sections were overexposed to the acid-alcohol solution used for decolorization.

• Staining solution was used at room temperature instead of heated when using the Ziehl-Neelsen method.

SOLUTIONS:

• Decrease time in the acid-alcohol solution or use a weaker solution.

• Repeat staining with heated carbolfuchsin solution and decolorize again.

COMMENTS: The amount of acid used in the decolorizing solution can lead to variable staining. Weak-staining organisms can be decolorized by overtreatment with

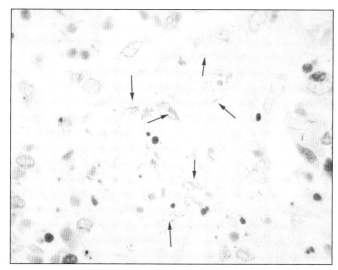

Figure 6.7. The organisms present in this Ziehl-Neelsen–stained section have been over-decolorized and, rather than staining bright red, are indistinct and dull, even though the background is clear. Organisms are present at the arrows.

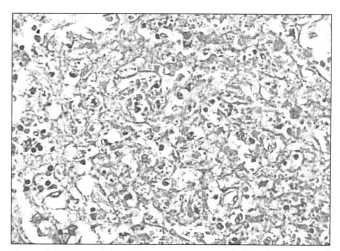

Figure 6.8. The methylene blue counterstain is too dark in this section. Cell nuclei are completely darkened. The connective tissue is dark blue. The organisms present have absorbed the counterstain to the extent that they have turned purple rather than bright red.

acid-alcohol or by failing to heat the carbolfuchsin. There is a fine line between not enough time and too much time in the decolorizing solution used in most acid-fast procedures. Generally speaking, most acid-fast bacteria are fairly resistant to being over-decolorized. However, when organisms die, their fatty capsule is compromised along with their acid-fast properties. The carbohydrate component of the organism can then be demonstrated with a methenamine silver or periodic acid–Schiff (PAS) reaction.[17]

PROBLEM: Counterstain Is Too Dark

APPEARANCE: The counterstain used is too dark, staining all cells and structures in the background. There is reduced contrast between the red acid-fast organisms and the background, obscuring or changing the color of the organisms (Figures 6.8 and 6.9).

CAUSES:

- Sections were exposed too long to methylene blue, light green, or fast green FCF counterstain.
- Counterstain solution was not properly prepared.

SOLUTIONS:

- Reduce the time in the counterstain solution.
- Acidify the counterstain by diluting dye into 0.5% to 1% acetic acid.

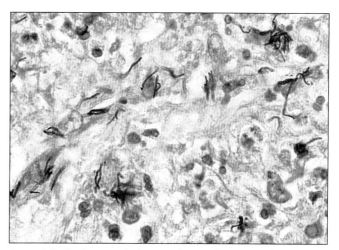

Figure 6.9. This figure is a higher magnification of Figure 6.8, showing purple organisms along with overstained cell nuclei and connective tissue.

- Differentiate or lighten the counterstain by longer treatment in water and alcohols after staining.
- Remake counterstain solution.

COMMENT: In a well-stained section, the counterstain should color only the nuclei of the cells in the background.

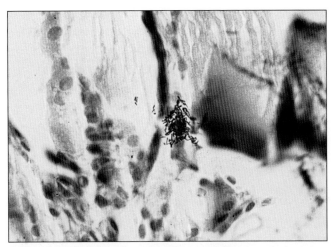

Figure 6.10. A distinctive clump of acid-fast organisms is above the focal plane of the section in this figure. They are probably a tap water contaminant.

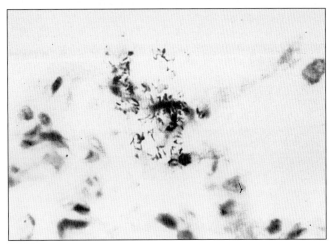

Figure 6.11. In this example of acid-fast contaminants, the organisms overlay the cells and are not in the focal plane.

PROBLEM: False-Positive Staining Caused by Contamination

APPEARANCE: If present, the contaminant usually appears as clumps or "floaters" above the focal plane of the section (Figures 6.10 and 6.11).

CAUSES:

- Growth of acid-fast organisms has occurred in tap water lines and tubing.
- Flotation bath surface has become contaminated from using tap water.

SOLUTIONS:

- Always use a known positive control as well as a negative control slide cut from the same day's workload.
- Use Millipore-filtered water before the carbolfuchsin step and for the first rinse after the stain.

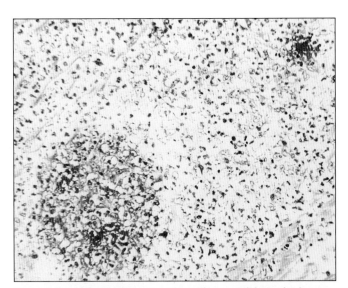

Figure 6.12. Carbolfuchsin was not adequately removed during decolorization of this Fite control section because of inadequate blotting of the mineral oil–xylene solution used in deparaffinization. Acid-fast organisms, which are obvious in the center of the section, are obscured by the remaining oily spots.

COMMENTS: Acid-fast organisms have been reported in common tap water, growing in tap water lines and in distilled water reservoirs. Caution should be observed on a daily basis. However, it may not be practical to use only Millipore-filtered water for AFB stains, as has been suggested.[18,19] The use of known positive and known negative tissue controls cut from the same clean water bath can virtually eliminate the possibility of a false-positive stain being interpreted incorrectly. It is especially important that the negative control sections and the patient's tissue be cut and floated on the same water bath. AFB contaminants from extrinsic water sources may appear on the slide above or outside the focal plane of the section. Contaminants from the surface of the water bath may appear below the focal plane of the section; this type may pose a serious diagnostic problem.

PROBLEM: Blotchy, Nonspecific Staining With the Fite Method

APPEARANCE: Some areas appear to stain properly, while other areas appear to either not stain at all or are not properly decolorized and thus have spotty, blotchy staining (Figures 6.12 and 6.13).

CAUSE:

- There was a failure to adequately blot and remove or loosen the mineral oil or peanut oil used in deparaffinization.

SOLUTIONS:

- After deparaffinization, blot section thoroughly with a soft, oil-absorbent paper or cloth.

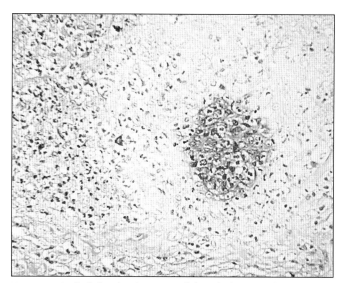

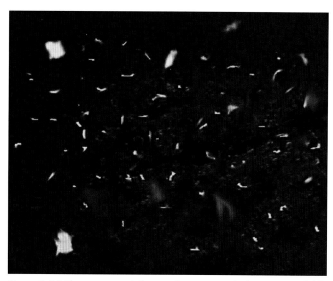

Figure 6.13. The light-colored ring around the red oily spot in the right center of this section represents a barrier created by inadequate blotting of the mineral oil–xylene solution. Acid-fast organisms are present at the margin of the light area but are obscured beneath it.

Figure 6.14. There are several objects in this auramine-rhodamine–stained slide that are not consistent with the expected size and shape of mycobacteria. There are several other objects that appear fuzzy and indistinct. The reviewer must use strict morphologic criteria to assess for bacteria.

- Rinse well in moderately warm water to further loosen the oils.

- Using a microwave or water bath, thoroughly heat the carbolfuchsin solution used for staining. Dip the sections in the warm solution several times.

- Wash well in moderately warm water after staining in carbolfuchsin.

COMMENTS: As previously mentioned, organisms such as *M leprae*, *Nocardia*, and *Cryptosporidium* are frequently completely decolorized by the standard Ziehl-Neelsen technique. The mineral oil or peanut oil mixtures used for deparaffinization in the Fite method appear to provide a protective coating around these partially acid-fast organisms, which helps to avoid subsequent over-decolorization. However, if the oils are not adequately removed with blotting and a short warm-water rinse before exposure to the carbolfuchsin solution, blotchy and irregular staining may result. These oils resist penetration by the carbolfuchsin, essentially forming a barrier over the section.

PROBLEM: Nonspecific Staining With Fluorescent Methods

APPEARANCE: Objects that are not consistent with the shape, size, and overall morphology of mycobacteria exhibit the same color of fluorescence as the bacteria (Figure 6.14).

CAUSES:

- The stain solution was not filtered before use.

- There was repeated heating and cooling of the stain solution.

SOLUTIONS:

- Filter all stain solutions immediately before use.

- Avoid repeated heating and cooling of the stain solution.

COMMENTS: The stain solution used in this fluorescent technique will often become contaminated with clumps of the dye that deposit onto the slides during staining. Review of known positive controls should help familiarize the microscopist with the expected morphology of mycobacteria. To use this method, one must be familiar with the fluorescence microscope and its filters and optics.

References

1. Hawkin C, Gold K, Whimbey E, et al. Mycobacterium avium complex infections in patients with the acquired immunodeficiency syndrome. *Ann Intern Med.* 1986;105:184-188.

2. Carson FL. *Histotechnology: A Self-Instructional Text.* 2nd ed. Chicago, IL: American Society of Clinical Pathologists; 1997: 188-192.

3. Lillie R. *Histopathologic Technic and Practical Histochemistry.* 3rd ed. New York, NY: McGraw-Hill; 1965: 575-581.

4. Winn W. Current concepts in pathologic diagnosis: bacterial diseases. *J Histotechnol.* 1995;18(3):241.

5. Ellis R, Zabrowarny L. Safer staining method for acid fast bacilli. *J Clin Pathol.* 1993;46:559-560.

6. Cserni C. Elimination of phenol from the auramine fluorescence staining method for acid fast bacilli. *J Histotechnol.* 1998;21(3):241-242.

7. Wade HW. A modification of the Fite formaldehyde (Fite) method for staining acid-fast bacilli in paraffin sections. *Stain Technol.* 1957;32, 287.

8. Bancroft J, Stevens A. *Theory and Practice of Histological Techniques.* 2nd ed. New York, NY: Churchill Livingstone; 1982: 278-296.

9. Kuper SWA, May JR. Detection of acid-fast organisms in tissue sections by fluorescence microscopy. *J Pathol Bacteriol.* 1960;79:59.

10. Truant JP, Brett WA, Thomas W. Fluorescence microscopy of tubercle bacilli stained with auramine and rhodamine. *Henry Ford Hosp Med Bull.* 1962;10:287-296.

11. Elias, JM. Infectious organisms: meeting the new challenge in surgical pathology. *J Histotechnol.* 1995;18(3):177-178.

12. Churukian CJ. Demonstration of mycobacteria: a brief review with special emphasis on fluorochrome staining. *J Histotechnol.* 1991;14:117.

13. Fukunaga H, Murakami T, Gondo T, Sugi K, Ishihara T. Sensitivity of acid-fast staining for Mycobacterium tuberculosis in formalin-fixed tissue. *Am J Respir Crit Care Med.* 2002;166:994-997.

14. Minnikin DE, Minnikin SM, Parlett JH, Goodfellow M, Magnusson M. Mycolic acid patterns of some species of Mycobacterium. *Arch Microbiol.* 1984;139:225-231.

15. Fite GL, Fite CW. Dye adsorption by mycobacteria. *Int J Lepr.* 1965;33:324-341.

16. Cocito C. Biological, chemical, immunological and staining properties of bacteria isolated from tissues of leprosy patients. *Eur J Epidemiol.* 1985;1:202-231.

17. Wear DJ, Hadfield TL, Connor DH. Periodic acid-Schiff reaction stains Mycobacterium tuberculosis, Mycobacterium leprae, Mycobacterium ulcerans, Mycobacterium chelonei (abscesses) and Mycobacterium kansasii. *Arch Pathol Lab Med.* 1985; 109:701-703.

18. Carson F, Kingsley WB, Haberman S, Race GJ. Unclassified mycobacteria contamination acid-fast stains of tissue sections. *Tech Bull Regist Med Technol.* 1964;34:65-68.

19. Wang W. Contamination of tissue sections with acid-fast bacilli as detected by fluorescence microscopy. *Am J Clin Pathol.* 1969;51:71-75.

Robert L. Lott

Helicobacter pylori are curved or spiral-shaped bacteria found in the stomach and duodenum in a high percentage of patients with chronic gastritis and duodenal ulcer. The organism is most prevalent in the gastric antrum, but it also colonizes oxyntic and cardiac mucosa. The bacterium was initially named *Campylobacter pyloridis*, then *C pylori,* and in 1989, after DNA sequencing and other data showed that the bacterium did not belong in the *Campylobacter* genus, it was placed in its own genus, *Helicobacter*. More than 35 species of *Helicobacter* have now been described, but only a few have been shown to cause gastritis in humans, including *H pylori, H felis, H fennelliae, H cinaedi,* and *H heilmannii*. Among these, *H pylori* is the most common. Gastritis due to *H pylori* is associated with duodenal ulcer, gastric ulcer (less commonly), and gastric malignancies, including adenocarcinoma and lymphoma. The relative risk of these conditions varies greatly in different populations, presumably because of genetic factors.

H pylori can be seen in tissue sections with the routine hematoxylin and eosin (H&E) stain (Figure 7.1) on close examination at high magnification (400x). However, this method is less reliable than special stains when the organisms are scarce or difficult to recognize. Most laboratories use colorimetric, silver, or immunohistochem-istry (IHC) techniques to definitively demonstrate this bacterium. It is a gram-negative bacillus having the distinctive morphology of a stumpy, curved rod; however, staining with the conventional Gram technique gives inconsistent results. The size of the organisms in the stained section is dependent upon the stain employed. With silver impregnation techniques, the organism appears thick and can be readily identified without oil immersion (400x magnification). On the other hand, the Giemsa procedure stains only the inner portion of the organism, making it appear thinner and more difficult to distinguish.[1] Many unique, special staining techniques have been developed, and some older methods have been modified for the histological assessment of *H pylori*; however, all have some defects from the standpoint of sensitivity, convenience, stability, visibility of the organisms, or cost. These different methods, presented in Table 7.1, are discussed below.

The Simple Blue Stains

The first group of these stains may be termed the "simple blue" stains, such as toluidine blue, methylene blue, cresyl echt violet, and Diff-Quik® (or the "modified" Giemsa). These stains, consisting of single basic dye solutions, can be performed rapidly and are very cost effective, but because the bacteria and all other cellular components are stained various shades of the same color (blue), contrast between the two is rarely optimal. A careful search is required to identify organisms if they are not present in large numbers. Thin sections (3 μm) show the organisms best. Reproducibility in this group of stains, however, is good, and because of their simplicity, these techniques are easily automated on modern stainers used for routine H&E stains.

Toluidine blue stains have been used in the histology laboratory for years. When used at an acid pH (3.2 or below), toluidine blue stains sulfated mucocompounds, such as mast cell granules, metachromatically. At a more neutral pH (6.6 to 7.0), it stains bacteria dark blue and other tissue elements varying intensities of blue.[2] A very dilute solution of the dye, typically 0.01%, is used when staining for bacteria.

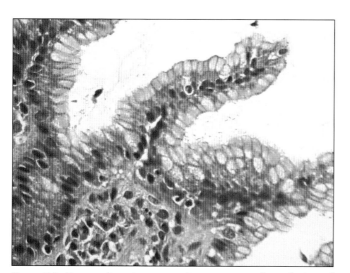

Figure 7.1. Hematoxylin and eosin stain demonstrates *H pylori* at the luminal surface. The bacteria are basophilic, staining light blue-black with hematoxylin.

Table 7.1. Comparison of Techniques for the Identification of *Helicobacter pylori*

Stain (Reference) by Group	Interobserver Agreement	Relative Cost	Average Time/Slide	Specificity	Reproducibility of Technique
Hematoxylin and Eosin	Moderate	Cheap	20–25 min	Moderate	High
Simple Blue Stains					
Toluidine blue	Moderate	Cheapest	4–6 min	Moderate – High	High
Modified Giemsa (Diff-Quik II)	High	Cheapest	4–6 min	Moderate – High	Very High
Cresyl echt violet	High	Cheap	12–15 min	Moderate – High	High
Histochemical Stains					
Leung (Alcian yellow/toluidine blue)	High	Moderate	25–30 min	High	High
Gimenez	Moderate	Moderate	10–15 min	Moderate	Good
Sayeed	Moderate	Moderate	15–20 min	Moderate	Good
True Giemsa Stains					
Wright-Giemsa	High	Cheap	10–15 min	Moderate – High	Good
Jenner-Giemsa	High	Moderate	45–60 min	Moderate – High	Good
May Grünwald Giemsa	High	Moderate	45–60 min	Moderate – High	Good
Silver Stains					
Warthin-Starry	High	Expensive	35–45 min	High	Poor – Good
Modified Steiner	High	Expensive	35–45 min	High	Poor – Good
H pylori silver stain (HpSS)	Moderate	Expensive	30–40 min	High	Poor – Good
Combination Stains					
Genta	Moderate	Expensive	60–80 min	High	Poor – Good
El-Zimaity	Moderate	Expensive	60–80 min	High	Poor – Good
HpSS	Moderate	Expensive	30–40 min	High	Poor – Good
Immunohistochemistry	Highest	Expensive	2–3.5 h	Highest	Very High

The Diff-Quik stain,[3,4] or the Diff-Quik II solution used alone,[5] has found particular favor with many pathologists and laboratories as an adjunct stain for identification of *H pylori*. The Diff-Quik stain, often referred to as the "modified" or "rapid" Giemsa, is a modification of the Wright stain used primarily in hematology. It consists of three solutions: a methanolic fixative and two aqueous dye solutions. The first dye, Solution I, is a buffered solution of Eosin Y, an anionic dye. The second dye, Solution II, is a proprietary mixture of the cationic thiazine dyes methylene blue and azure A in a water solution with a buffer. For hematologic applications, such as blood smears or touch-preparations, the technique is very rapid, taking only 15 to 20 seconds from beginning to end. However, for tissue sections, the times must be extended to about 2 to 3 minutes in each of the three solutions. There is no washing between steps.

Diff-Quik II or one of its generic equivalents, such as Hema 3 solution II, is used alone for staining *H pylori*. This procedure is very quick and economical, requiring only 1 to 2 minutes in the staining solution, and the reagent can be reused repeatedly. A small amount of differentiation is required for optimal contrast; however, a prolonged time in the water rinses or in the dehydrating alcohols will cause excess decolorization, making the organisms difficult to identify.

The cresyl echt violet method described by Gomes[6,7] is also very simple and fast. Bacteria are stained deep violet-purple and are very easy to locate. They contrast well against a light background. A tiny amount of glacial acetic acid (2 drops) in 50 mL of 95% alcohol is required to properly differentiate the cresyl echt violet. This method is inexpensive enough that it could be used routinely on all gastric and duodenal biopsies.[1]

Dye-Based Histochemical Stains

Over the last 10 years, a second group of moderately complex, dye-based histochemical techniques has emerged for detection of *H pylori*. Many pathologists prefer these methods because the bacteria are stained a different color from the background mucin and cell cytoplasm, which dramatically improves contrast and facilitates detection. Examples include the Leung, the Gimenez (and its modifications), and the Sayeed methods.

The Alcian yellow-toluidine blue (AY-TB) technique, first described by Leung in 1996,[8] has gained popularity because of high contrast between the stained organism and the background mucin. Carbohydrates present in the neutral mucin of the stomach lining are oxidized by periodic acid, treated with sodium metabisulfite, and stained with Alcian yellow. The bacteria and other tissue elements are stained varying intensities of blue. This method yields clear, crisp bacterial staining and good tissue morphology. The blue-stained organisms stand out very well against the yellow mucin and background and are easy to locate. The interpretation of the slide may be less time consuming than with other methods. Because of the scarcity of the Alcian yellow dye, an alternative procedure has been developed that mimics the results of the original Leung method.[9] This procedure and the reagent components are commercially available.

The Gimenez technique, first described in 1964 for detection of rickettsia,[10] uses basic fuchsin in an aqueous solution with phenol and ethanol (carbolfuchsin) to stain the bacteria red, magenta, or pink. A malachite green counterstain gives a blue-green cast to the surrounding tissue. It is a relatively simple technique that takes about 15 minutes to complete. The contrast between the red bacteria and the background makes screening of the slide easy.[11] However, many have found it difficult to obtain consistent results with this method. There have been reports that the carbolfuchsin reagent tends to precipitate; therefore, regular filtering may be required.[1]

The Sayeed stain for *H pylori*[12] is similar to the Leung method, but it uses Schiff reagent to color the mucin magenta and methylene blue to color the bacteria. Nuclei are stained with Mayer hematoxylin. Users have reported inconsistent results. The bacteria are often indistinct and "muddy" while superimposed on a red background. The poor contrast makes searching for the organisms both slow and tedious.[1] This method is not recommended for routine use.

True Giemsa Stains

Romanowsky-type Giemsa techniques are excellent for the demonstration of bacteria in tissue sections. This group of stains, not to be confused with the modified Giemsa (Diff-Quik), can be described as polychromatic because they are compound dyes or dye mixtures that contain components of different colors. The most common example used in histopathology is a combination of the basic dye methylene blue and the acidic dye eosin. The pH of the staining solution is important and ideally

should be adjusted for different fixatives. More acidic pH levels give more chromatin staining and less cytoplasmic basophilia; less acidic pH levels give denser nuclei and increased cytoplasmic basophilia. The pH level should be between 6.4 and 6.9. Numerous modifications of the Romanowsky methods have been described, particularly for application to tissue sections. In a well-done Giemsa stain, *H pylori* appear thin and distinctly blue. Bacterial shapes are easily recognizable and contrast very well because the mucin is essentially unstained. The staining obtained in tissue sections is more variable than in smears because the protocols used require additional steps (differentiation, dehydration, clearing), and tissue sections contain more stainable components.[13] Some stains are used in combination to produce the desired coloring of cell and tissue components, as with the Jenner-Giemsa and May Grünwald-Giemsa techniques.[14]

The Romanowsky methods used for tissue sections cannot be considered rapid techniques, taking 45 minutes to complete; however, they provide adequate staining of the bacteria, as well as excellent tissue morphology. Care must be taken not to overdifferentiate the stained slides. The lack of contrast after overdifferentiation makes it difficult to identify organisms even though mucin is unstained.

Silver Stains

Some laboratories find traditional and microwave-accelerated silver staining very effective for demonstrating *H pylori*, especially the Steiner technique and its modifications[15-17] and the Warthin-Starry methods.[18-20] These time-tested methods, however, are labor intensive, require multiple reagents with elaborate solution preparation, and require some expertise for optimal results. The literature is rich with modifications and helpful hints about how to achieve clearly delineated bacteria with minimal staining of the background and connective tissue. However, anyone who has performed these techniques is familiar with just how capricious they can be. Use of freshly prepared sensitizing and silver solutions for impregnation is vital. Many of the microwave modifications call for heating the impregnating silver solution to very high temperatures (in excess of 80° to 90°C). If the solution is not freshly prepared, overheating may cause it to break down, generating random, nonspecific deposition of silver granules onto the section and slide. The reducing solution or developer must contain freshly prepared hydroquinone and a small amount of silver nitrate for adequate visualization of organisms.

The correct percentage and quantity of each reagent in the all-important reducing step should be carefully calculated and measured each time the procedure is performed. Finally, a balance has to be achieved between

Table 7.2. Comparison of Silver Staining Methods for *Helicobacter pylori*

Method	Steiner	Warthin-Starry	Dieterle
Sensitizer	0.1–1.0% Uranyl nitrate *0.01% Phosphotungstic acid *10% Zinc formalin *1.0% Lead nitrate solution *0.5% Lead nitrate–Gum mastic	None (for *Helicobacter*)	1.0% Uranyl nitrate
Impregnating Solution	*0.1–1.0% Silver nitrate (with heat)	*0.5–1.0% Silver nitrate (with heat)	1% Silver nitrate (with heat)
Reducing Solution	2.5% Gum mastic – 15 mL 1.0% hydroquinone – 25 mL 1% Silver nitrate – 0.27 mL	2% Silver nitrate – 9.0 mL 5% Gelatin – 22.5 mL 0.15% Hydroquinone – 12.0 mL	Hydroquinone – 0.75 g Sodium sulfite – 0.15 g 37% Formaldehyde – 5 mL Acetone – 5 mL Pyridine – 5 mL Distilled water – 30 mL 10% Gum mastic – 5 mL

* Published modifications

underdevelopment, which results in pale-staining organisms against a pale or clear background, and overdevelopment, which results in thick, black organisms against a dark yellow-brown background. To the naked eye, an underdeveloped section is pale yellow, and an overdeveloped section is dark golden brown. To achieve the proper balance, the use of more than one section of patient tissue and paired control slide may be the best course of action, removing them at different times during the reduction. The choice of method appears to be a matter of preference based upon satisfactory performance and reproducibility. As with all silver staining methods, strict adherence to the laboratory-validated protocol and control of the required time and temperature variables cannot be overemphasized.

The replacement of the uranyl nitrate solution with lead nitrate,[21] zinc-formalin,[22] or phosphotungstic acid[23] has been advocated to address the potential radioactive hazard involved in the use of uranyl nitrate.[24] In a large, two-part study by Buesa,[23] which tested multiple sensitizers at various dilutions in an effort to find a suitable replacement for uranyl nitrate in the Steiner method, only 0.01% phosphotungstic acid proved to be as consistently reliable as uranyl nitrate for the detection of *H pylori*.

The Warthin-Starry method and its modifications are a popular alternative technique because the uranyl nitrate step is not necessary except when staining for spirochetes. It may be the simplest of all the silver staining methods for *H pylori*, but it can be inconsistent and contains rather strict pH and temperature requirements. Organisms usually stain a more intense black with the Warthin-Starry method, but background staining is more pronounced than with the Steiner or Dieterle techniques.[20] Nuclei will stain an intense brown, and connective tissues varying shades of brown. Many histotechnologists have found the method to be difficult. Recently, however, an automated, special staining platform has been marketed that uses unique patented reagents and standardized conditions; this platform has optimized the Warthin-Starry stain, making it consistently reproducible. A comparison of silver methods used for *H pylori* along with their published modifications is found in Table 7.2.

Combination Stains

The Genta triple stain[25] and the more recently described El-Zimaity triple method[26] combine the Steiner silver impregnation with Alcian blue, pH 2.5, and H&E. They are popular with gastrointestinal pathologists because they highlight small foci of intestinal metaplasia (Alcian blue positive) while simultaneously demonstrating *Helicobacter* and tissue morphology. The use of uranyl nitrate in the Steiner element of the Genta technique prompted the El-Zimaity group to substitute a lead nitrate-gum mastic solution in the sensitization step.

In 1997, the novel *Helicobacter pylori* silver stain (HpSS)[27] was proposed, which utilizes the argyrophilic nucleolar organizing region (AgNOR) reaction. Sections are impregnated with hot silver nitrate, followed by the AgNOR silver solution. After development in the dark to visualize the *H pylori* organisms, the sections are toned or cleared with a unique "blue toning" solution. H&E counterstaining provides for simultaneous assessment of organisms and tissue morphology. The sensitivity of this technique is excellent; however, *H heilmanii* and other non-*H pylori* bacteria are also stained with this technique.

Immunohistochemical Stains

Immunohistochemistry (IHC) for detection of *H pylori* was first introduced in the late 1980s[28-30] and has become invaluable for difficult cases. Modern pathology laboratories that perform IHC studies routinely have found that the availability of quality antibodies, improved biotin-free detection reagents, and automation has made this methodology both easy and moderately affordable. As with any IHC test for an infectious agent, rigorous testing and validation is needed to optimize the assay and understand the potential for cross-reactivity with other species. However, many studies have confirmed IHC as the true "gold standard" in terms of both sensitivity and specificity for detection of *H pylori*.[27,31-35] IHC is particularly useful for the identification of the coccoid forms of *H pylori*, which are difficult to recognize with any other staining technique.[36]

Many laboratories use IHC as a tool to identify *H pylori* in biopsies previously examined by H&E that show the typical pattern of inflammation associated with *H pylori* gastritis. These cases may include those in which dye-based stains for the organisms have been performed but were inconclusive. In almost all studies comparing methods of detection, including colorimetric, silver, and IHC, interobserver agreement was highest for IHC; however, most agree that it is too expensive and time consuming to be used as an initial screen.

Discussion

So which special stain is best for detection of *H pylori* in sections of gastric/antral/duodenal biopsies? There seems to be no simple answer to this question. The H&E stain alone may be entirely adequate for most cases. It is a well-tested, inexpensive, and simple staining method, requiring a relatively short period of time to perform, with highly reproducible results.[37] It has the added advantage of enabling simultaneous assessment of morphological changes accompanying *H pylori* infection.

Some laboratories favor the "modified Giemsa" stain for its simplicity alone. Others argue that a stain with more contrast, such as the Alcian yellow-toluidine blue,

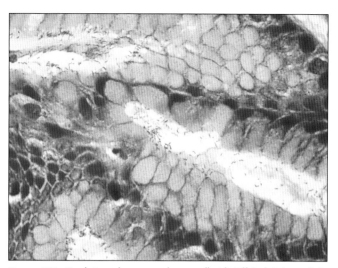

Figure 7.2. *H pylori* are demonstrated very well with Diff-Quik Solution II. In a well-stained section, the bacteria are dark blue against a pale blue-green background.

is best.[38] IHC is particularly useful in cases where inflammation is limited and the number of organisms is small. When the organisms are present, careful examination, usually on high power (40x objective) will almost always reveal them, whichever stain is used.

Controls

Tissue known to contain moderate numbers of *H pylori* bacteria must be used with any of the staining techniques. Control material for the procedure can usually be obtained by reviewing prior gastric resections for chronic gastritis or peptic ulcer. In gastric biopsies, the organisms are normally found on the epithelial surface or in the mucosal glandular folds. Positive biopsies can be used for control material. It is recommended that a positive control slide always be included so that the relative color balance of organisms with respect to the background can be assessed.

What Should Be Seen in a Good Stain for *Helicobacter*

Regardless of the method used, the organisms should contrast well with the background structures. With the simple blue stains, the bacteria should stain dark blue against a lighter blue background. With the histochemical stains, organisms are stained one color against a background of a different color. The "true" Giemsa stains color the organism blue against a colorless background. Silver-stained *Helicobacter* should be distinctly black against a yellowish-tan to light brown background. Organisms stained using IHC techniques are either brown or red, depending on the enzyme-chromagen combination used. *Helicobacter* stained with an H&E stain is seen in Figure 7.1. Examples of good special stains for *Helicobacter* are seen in Figures 7.2 through 7.9.

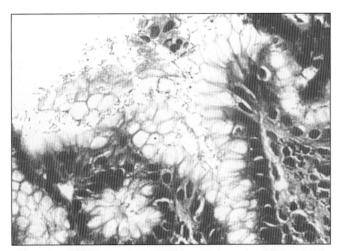

Figure 7.3. Numerous purple-blue bacteria are seen on the surface and in the lumen of the glands in this antral biopsy stained with the cresyl echt violet method.

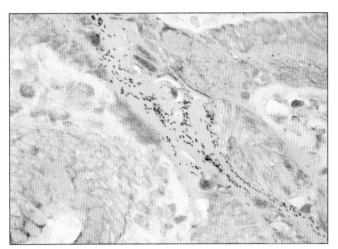

Figure 7.4. The popular histochemical stain Alcian yellow–toluidine blue demonstrates well-differentiated blue bacteria against a background of yellow mucus.

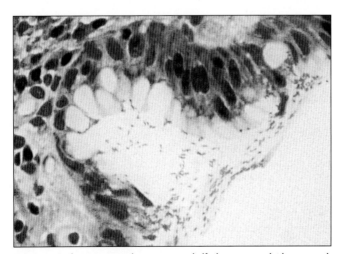

Figure 7.5. The Gimenez technique uses carbolfuchsin to stain the bacteria red, magenta, or pink. The malachite green counterstain gives a blue-green background cast to the surrounding tissue.

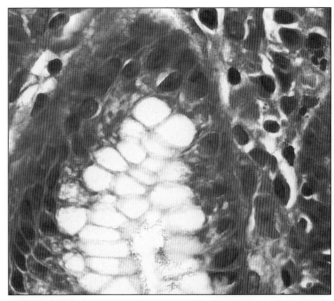

Figure 7.6. This Giemsa stain demonstrates *H pylori* organisms that are easily recognized against the clear to light-blue epithelial mucin.

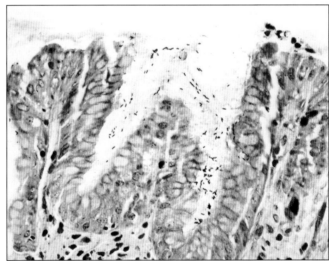

Figure 7.7. *H pylori* are well stained using an automated special stain platform and the Warthin-Starry silver stain. (Photo courtesy of David R. Kelly, MD and Rita Humphrey, HT(ASCP), Children's Hospital, Birmingham, Alabama.)

Problems Encountered With Stains for *Helicobacter pylori*

PROBLEM: Lack of Contrast With Simple Blue, Diff-Quik, Histochemical, and Giemsa Methods

APPEARANCE: Organisms are indistinct and lack contrast with background structures (Figures 7.10 through 7.14).

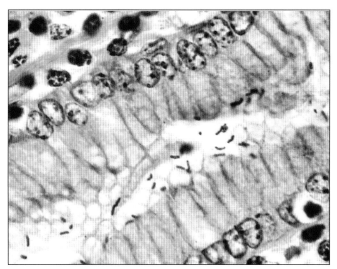

Figure 7.8. The Genta triple stain is used to label intestinal metaplasia (Alcian blue positive), while simultaneously demonstrating *H pylori* and biopsy morphology.

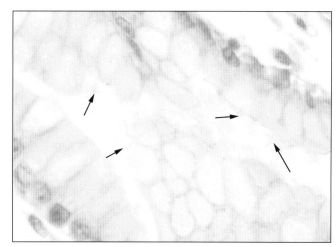

Figure 7.10. This Diff-Quik Solution II-stained section has been almost completely decolorized in alcohol before coverslipping. The organisms (at arrows) lack contrast and are essentially the same color as the background epithelium and mucin. (Compare with Figure 7.2.)

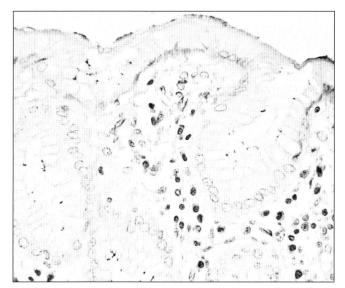

Figure 7.9. Immunohistochemistry is a very sensitive and specific technique for the detection of *H pylori* in tissue sections. It is particularly useful for the identification of the coccoid forms, which are difficult to recognize with any other staining technique.

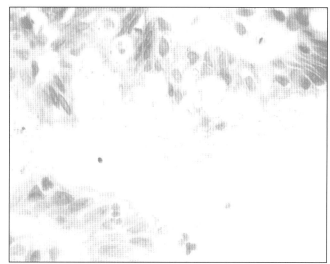

Figure 7.11. This section, stained with the cresyl echt violet method, has been overdifferentiated in alcoholic acetic acid. The *H pylori* bacteria have lost most of their characteristic purple color and do not contrast well with the background. (Compare with Figure 7.3.)

CAUSES:

- Stained sections have been overdifferentiated, usually in alcohol or acetic washes.
- Stained sections have spent prolonged time in the distilled water rinse or in the dehydrating alcohols at the end of the method.

SOLUTIONS:

- There should be strict adherence to validated staining protocol (times, washing, differentiation, etc).

- Quickly wash, dehydrate, and clear slides at the end of the method.

COMMENTS: Care must be taken not to overdifferentiate the stained slides. One of the most common mistakes with these methods is to leave the finished slides in the dehydrating alcohols at the end of the method before clearing and coverslipping.

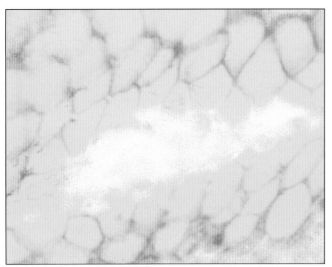

Figure 7.12. The *H pylori* bacteria present in this gastric gland are pale and indistinct. This section stained with Alcian yellow–toluidine blue was left in the dehydrating alcohols too long before clearing and coverslipping. (Compare with Figure 7.4.)

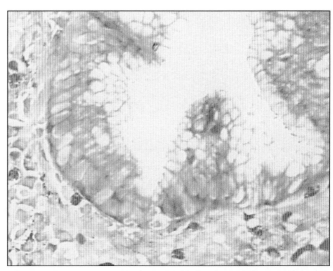

Figure 7.14. Bacteria present in this gastric gland lack contrast because of poor differentiation and overdehydration of this Giemsa stain. (Compare with Figure 7.6.)

PROBLEM: Understaining or Nonspecific Staining With Silver Impregnation Methods

APPEARANCE: Organisms are indistinct and lack contrast with background structures. Granular silver precipitate overlays the tissue section (Figures 7.15, 7.16, and 7.17).

CAUSES:

- Sections were not immersed long enough in silver impregnation solution.
- Silver impregnation solution was not adequately heated.
- Silver nitrate solutions were not freshly made.
- Silver impregnation solution was too hot.
- Tissue sections were either underexposed or overexposed to developing solutions.
- Developing solution contained too much hydroquinone or silver nitrate.

SOLUTIONS:

- Preheat silver impregnation solutions; check temperature and stir slides into both the silver impregnation solution and the developer and agitate. Use of a water bath is recommended.
- Best results are achieved if the silver solution is heated to between 60° and 70°C. Be careful if using microwave heating; water bath heating is highly reli-

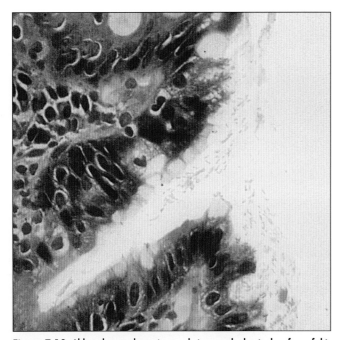

Figure 7.13. Although some bacteria are obvious on the luminal surface of this gastric biopsy, they have lost their characteristic red-pink color in this poorly differentiated Gimenez-stained section. (Compare with Figure 7.5.)

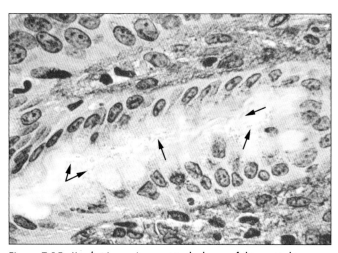

Figure 7.15. *H pylori* (arrows) present in the lumen of this gastric biopsy are very lightly stained. The organisms should be distinctly black and contrast well against the clear to-yellow-brown mucin and epithelial cell cytoplasm. (Compare with Figure 7.7.)

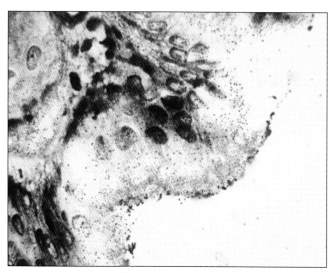

Figure 7.16. In this modified Steiner stain, a granular silver precipitate is deposited on the surface of the epithelium; this artifact is caused by overheating the silver impregnation solution. No morphologically consistent bacterial forms can be identified.

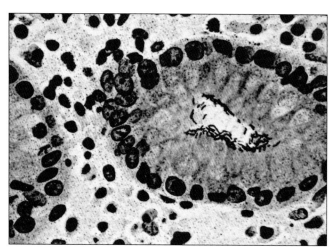

Figure 7.17. The *H pylori* organisms present in the lumen of this gland are well stained with the Genta method. Alcian blue staining reveals intestinal metaplasia. However, there is a distinct, fine, granular silver precipitate overlaying cells, stroma, and nuclei; this artifact is caused by overheating the silver impregnation solution.

able and recommended if performing the technique manually.

- Monitor color development of the section by checking slides at regular intervals (eg, 3, 6, 9, and 12 minutes).

- Use multiple sections of the same block, each with matched controls, and remove them from the developer at different times.

- Assure that the developing solution is properly made according to exact specifications of the technique being used.

- Use freshly prepared reagents and "clean" technique for each step of the protocol.

COMMENTS: Strict attention to detail and accurate formulation of the reducing solution is essential in achieving optimal contrast between the organisms and the background. Monitoring of development times and using multiple sections and multiple slides as described cannot be overemphasized; however, some tissue components can be expected to stain darkly even when the technique is correctly performed. Proper formulation and use of the reducing solution can alleviate many problems. It has been demonstrated that the concentrations of hydroquinone and silver in the developing solution are critical in avoiding background staining. Underdeveloped stains can be returned to the developing solution to deepen the color of the organisms and provide better contrast.

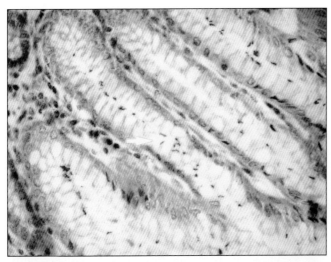

Figure 7.18. Within the lumen of this gastric resection specimen, bacteria that are morphologically consistent with *H pylori* are well stained, perhaps overstained. Epithelial cell cytoplasm, as well as inflammatory cells within the lamina propria, are staining with equal intensity. This type of nonspecific staining is unacceptable when staining for microorganisms.

PROBLEM: Nonspecific Staining in Sections Stained Using Immunohistochemistry
(See chapter 16 for additional problem-solving discussions regarding the use of IHC methods.)

APPEARANCE: Organisms are well stained, but structures other than the target bacteria are also stained. There is nonspecific staining of the patient's tissue coupled with an overstained positive control (Figure 7.18).

CAUSES:

- Concentration of the primary antibody is too strong.
- Diluted antibody has aged and broken down.
- Diluted antibody has been contaminated.
- Tissue sections are too thick.

SOLUTIONS:

- Check dilution of antibody, and repeat the staining procedure using freshly prepared antibody. Laboratory errors or use of uncalibrated pipettes can result in inaccurate dilutions being prepared.

- Re-titer primary antibody using at least three consecutive dilutions, and repeat validation process on control tissues. Antibodies differ in concentration from lot to lot and require validation before use.

- Cut all sections at the same thickness as the section used to validate antibody dilution. Thick sections can result in the localization of more antibody and result in concentrated staining.

COMMENTS: Nonspecific staining is one of the most common problems when using IHC methods for detecting and identifying microorganisms. The staining methodology must be rigorously tested and the method validated using multiple control section blocks. It is of vital importance that only the "target" antigen stains when performing IHC staining for *H pylori*.

References

1. Ratigan-Drexler K. A comparison of staining methods for Helicobacter pylori. *HistoLogic.* 1999;30:3-8.

2. Histotechnology Technical Methods. Stain for Helicobacter pylori. Toluidine Blue in Sorensons pH 6.8 Buffer. University of Nottingham Medical School Division of Histopathology; 1997. Available at: http://www.nottingham.ac.uk/pathology/protocols/tolbluehelm.html. Accessed January 20, 2009.

3. Gray SF, Wyatt JI, Rathbone BJ. Simplified techniques for identifying Campylobacter pyloridis. *J Clin Pathol.* 1986;39(11):1279.

4. Skipper R, DeStephano DB. A rapid stain for Campylobacter pylori in gastrointestinal sections using Diff-Quik. *J Histotechnol.* 1989;12:303-304.

5. Potvin CA. A modified Diff-Quik stain for Helicobacter pylori in gastrointestinal biopsies. *Lab Med.* 1994;25:389-391.

6. Burnett RA, Brown IL, Findlay J. Cresyl fast violet staining method for Campylobacter like organisms. *J Clin Pathol.* 1987; 40(3):353.

7. Gomes C. Rapid cresyl echt violet staining method for identifying Helicobacter pylori. *On Stage, NY State Histotechnological Society.* 1993;16(2):29.

8. Leung JK, Gibbon KJ, Vartanian RK. Rapid staining method for Helicobacter pylori in gastric biopsies. *J Histotechnol.* 1996;19:131-132.

9. Dapson D. New stains for Helicobacter pylori to replace alcian yellow and toluidine blue. *J Histotechnol.* 2002; 25(3):131-135.

10. Gimenez D.F. Staining Rickettsia in yolk-sac cultures. *Stain Technol.* 1964;39:135-140.

11. McMullen L, Walker MM, Bain LA, Karim QN, Baron JH. Histological identification of Campylobacter using Gimenez technique in gastric antral mucosa. *J Clin Pathol.* 1987;40(4):464-465.

12. Cohen LF, Sayeeduddin M, Phillips C, Shahab I. A new staining method for identification of Helicobacter pylori and simultaneous visualization of gastric morphologic features [published correction appears in Mod Pathol. 1998;11(1):18]. *Mod Pathol.* 1997;10(11):1160-1163.

13. Wittekind D, Schulte E, Schmidt G, Frank G. The standard Romanowsky-Giemsa stain in histology. *Biotech Histochem.* 1991;66:282-295.

14. Inwood MJ, Thomson S. Hematology and blood bank. In: Raphael SS, Lynch MJ, eds. *Lynch's Medical Laboratory Technology.* Vol. 2. 3rd ed. Philadelphia, PA: WB Saunders; 1976: 244-245.

15. Swisher LS. Modified Steiner procedure for microwave staining of spirochetes and nonfilamentous bacteria. *J Histotechnol.* 1987;10:241-243.

16. Churukian CJ, Garvey W. Microwave Steiner method for spirochetes and bacteria. *J Histotechnol.* 1990;13(1):45-47.

17. Garvey W, Fathi A, Bigelow F, Wynnchuk M. Revised modified Steiner to enhance visibility of spirochetes. *J Histotechnol.* 1995;18:57-60.

18. Faulkner RR, Lillie RD. A buffer modification of the Warthin-Starry silver method for spirochetes in single paraffin sections. *Stain Technol.* 1945;20(3):8l-82.

19. Vail KF. The Warthin-Starry impregnation technique with the microwave oven. *HistoLogic.* 1987;17:235-236.

20. Churukian CJ, Schenk EA. A Warthin-Starry method for spirochetes and bacteria using a microwave oven. *J Histotechnol.* 1988;11(3):149-151.

21. Elias JM, Green C. Modified Steiner method for the demonstration of spirochetes in tissue. *Am J Clin Pathol.* 1979;71:109-111.

22. Margeson LS, Chapman CM. Use of zinc formalin as a sensitizer in silver stains for spirochetes. *J Histotechnol.* 1996;19:135-138.

23. Buesa, RJ. Phosphotungstic acid eliminates uranyl nitrate as a sensitizer before the silver impregnation of Helicobacter pylori. *J Histotechnol.* 2001;24:113-116.

24. Darley JJ, Hisanori E. Potential hazards of uranium and its compounds in electron microscopy: a brief review. *J Microsc.* 1976;106:85-86.

25. Genta RM, Robason GO, Graham DY. Simultaneous visualization of Helicobacter pylori and gastric morphology: a new stain. *Hum Pathol.* 1994;25:221-226.

26. El-Zimaity HMT, Wu J, Graham DY. Modified Genta triple stain for identifying Helicobacter pylori. *J Clin Pathol.* 1999;52:693-694.

27. Doglioni C, Turrin M, Macrì E, Chiarelli C, Germana B, Barbareschi M: HpSS: a new silver staining method for Helicobacter pylori. *Clin Pathol.* 1997; 50(6):461-464.

28. Barbosa A, Queiroz DM, Mendes EN, Rocha GA, Lima GF, Oliveira CA. Immunocytochemical identification of Campylobacter pylori in gastritis and correlation with culture. *Arch Pathol Lab Med.* 1988;112:523-525.

29. Negrini R, Lisato L, Cavazzini P, et al. Monoclonal antibodies for specific immunoperoxidase detection of Campylobacter pylori. *Gastroenterology.* 1989; 96:414-420.

30. Cartun RW, Kryzmowski GA, Pederson CA, Morin SG, Van Kruiningen HI, Berman MM. Immunocytochemical identification of Helicobacter pylori in formalin-fixed gastric biopsies. *Mod Pathol.* 1991; 4:498-502.

31. Toulaymat M, Marconi S, Garb J, Otis C, Nash S. Endoscopic biopsy pathology of Helicobacter pylori gastritis: comparison of bacterial detection by immunohistochemistry and Genta stain. *Arch Pathol Lab Med.* 1999;123:778-781.

32. Jonkers D, Stobberingh E, de Bruine A, Arends JW, Stockbrügger R. Evaluation of immunohistochemistry for the detection of Helicobacter pylori in gastric mucosal biopsies. *J Infect.* 1997;35(2):149-154.

33. Ashton-Key M, Diss TC, Isaacson PG. Detection of Helicobacter pylori in gastric biopsy and resection specimens. *J Clin Pathol.* 1996;49(2):107-111.

34. Jhala N, Lechago S, Lechago J, Younes M. Is immunostaining for Helicobacter pylori superior to the special stain thiazine in detecting small numbers of H. pylori in gastric biopsies? *Appl Immunohistochem Mol Morphol.* 2002;10(1):82-84.

35. Kacar F, Culhaci N, Yükselen V, Meteoglu I, Dikicioglu E, Levi E. Histologic demonstration of Helicobacter pylori in gastric biopsies: which is the best staining method? *The Internet Journal of Pathology.* 2004;Vol. 3(1).

36. Marzio L, Angelucci D, Grossi L, Diodoro MG, Di Campli E, Cellini L. Anti-Helicobacter pylori specific antibody immunohistochemistry improves the diagnostic accuracy of Helicobacter pylori in biopsy specimen from patients treated with triple therapy. *Am J Gastroenterol.* 1998;93:223-226.

37. Anim JT, Al-Sobkie N, Prasad A, John B, Sharma PN, Al-Hamar I. Assessment of different methods for staining Helicobacter pylori in endoscopic gastric biopsies. *Acta Histochem.* 2000;102(2):29-137.

38. Rotimi O, Cairns A, Gray S, Moayyedi P, Dixon MF. Histological identification of Helicobacter pylori: comparison of staining methods. *J Clin Pathol.* 2000;53:756-759.

Spirochetes

Robert L. Lott

Spirochetes are long, very thin, helical, motile bacteria. Their name is derived from the Greek words for "coiled hair." The father of microbiology, Antonie van Leeuwenhoek, first sketched an oral spirochete, later named *Treponema denticola*, after viewing it through his primitive microscope in the 1670s. Despite their overall cell wall structure being that of gram-negative bacteria, spirochetes have unique cell morphology. The outer lipid membrane is typical of gram-negative bacteria, but the arrangement of structures inside this membrane is unique to the spirochetes. Inside is a "helical cell body." The helical body wraps around a central axis filled with proteinaceous filaments that resemble flagella and are called *axial filaments* or *endoflagella*. They are the locomotory organelles. Although classified as gram-negative bacteria, spirochetes stain very poorly or not at all with the Gram technique.

There is some diversity of size among the spirochetes. The larger species can be 25 μm long and some are only 0.075 μm in diameter. However, most spirochetes range between 0.10 and 0.15 μm in width and between 6 and 10 μm in length. In comparison, other bacteria, like most cocci, are 0.5 to 1.0 μm in diameter, and a single bacillus is typically 0.5 to 1.0 μm wide and from 1 to 4 μm long.

Because spirochetes are essentially non-Gram reactive and very thin, silver impregnation stains such as the Steiner, Warthin-Starry, and Dieterle procedures are required to demonstrate them (eg, *Treponema pallidum*, *Borrelia burgdorferi*, *Leptospira* species, *Bartonella* species, and *Calymmatobacterium granulomatis*). The most important member of the group is *Treponema pallidum*, the causative organism of syphilis. It may be found in variable numbers in the primary chancre, the initial lesion of infection.[1] Organisms are present in largest numbers in the secondary stage of syphilis, when they may be found in excised enlarged lymph nodes, biopsied oral ulcers, and genital condylomata. *T pallidum* is present in large numbers in the livers of some infants dying of congenital syphilis. Although rare in the United States, several diseases caused by organisms related to *T pallidum* are bejel (endemic syphilis); pinta, caused by *T carateum*; and yaws, caused by *T pertenue*. All are nonvenereal conditions caused by poor hygiene or spread via direct contact through skin lesions.

Other spirochetes of interest include the organism *Leptospira interrogans*, which causes a rare type of infective jaundice called leptospirosis or Weil's disease. These organisms can sometimes be demonstrated in the liver but are more common in animals than in humans. Another is the spirochete *Borrelia burgdorferi*, one of the largest spirochetes (0.3 x 25 μm) and the causative agent of the tick-borne infection Lyme disease. Silver stains may be sufficient for demonstration, but the organism is usually rare. Unless serial sections are stained and the technologist is experienced in recognizing positively stained organisms, the risk of a false-negative result is significant. Currently, the polymerase chain reaction (PCR), using solubilized tissue sections obtained from multiple levels of a paraffin block, is considered the best approach for detection of *B burgdorferi*.[2]

Immunohistochemistry, a sensitive and specific technology already in use in many laboratories, can easily be adapted to the search for spirochetes. Monoclonal and polyclonal antibodies to species of *Treponema*, *Leptospira*, and *Borrelia* are commercially available; however, these

Table 8.1. Spriochetal Infections

Pathogenic Spirochete	Human Disease	Vector/ Source
Borrelia		
B burgdorferi	Lyme disease	Ixodid ticks
B recurrentis	Epidemic relapsing fever	Body louse
B turicatae	Endemic relapsing fever	Ornithodoros ticks
Leptospira		
L interrogans	Leptospirosis (Weil's)	Contaminated animal urine
Treponema		
T pallidum	Syphilis	Sexual contact, transplacental
T pallidum ssp endemicum	Bejel (endemic syphilis)	Direct contact, contaminate eating utensils
T pallidum ssp pertenue	Yaws	Direct contact with infected skin lesions
T carateum	Pinta	

ssp = subspecies

Table 8.2. Comparison of Silver Staining Techniques for Spirochetes

Method	Steiner	Warthin-Starry	Dieterle
Sensitizer	0.1–1.0% Uranyl nitrate *0.01% Phosphotungstic acid *10% Zinc formalin *1.0% Lead nitrate solution *0.5% Lead nitrate–Gum mastic	None (for most bacteria, eg, *Helicobacter*) (Required for spirochetes) Non-gelling gelatin (Artisan)	1.0% Uranyl nitrate
Impregnating Solution	*0.1–1.0% Silver nitrate (with heat)	*0.5–1.0% Silver nitrate (with heat)	1% Silver nitrate (with heat)
Reducing Solution	2.5% Gum mastic – 15 mL 1.0% hydroquinone – 25 mL 1% Silver nitrate – 0.27 mL	2% Silver nitrate – 9.0 mL 5% Gelatin – 22.5 mL 0.15% Hydroquinone – 12.0 mL	Hydroquinone – 0.75 g Sodium sulfite – 0.15 g 37% Formaldehyde – 5 mL Acetone – 5 ml Pyridine – 5 mL Distilled water – 30 mL 10% Gum mastic – 5 mL

* Published modifications

antibodies must first undergo rigorous testing to identify cross-reactions with other bacterial organisms.[3] A list of spirochetes that cause human disease is found in Table 8.1

Early efforts to identify spirochetes in tissue include those of Levaditi[4] in 1905, who impregnated fixed tissue blocks with silver nitrate solutions in an effort to demonstrate *T pallidum*. In 1920, Warthin and Starry[5] and others published improvements to Levaditi's original concept and, along with Dieterle[6] in 1927, were the first to bring staining of spirochetes to individual tissue sections. Kerr offered an "improved Warthin-Starry method" in 1938 by adding pH requirements to the original technique.[7] Faulkner and Lillie later proposed other "buffer modifications."[8] Steiner and Steiner[9] introduced their "new simple silver stain" for bacteria and fungi in 1944, and many authors have worked with and published various modifications. In 1976, Van Orden and Greer used a modification of the Dieterle method to identify *Legionella pneumophilia* in tissue sections.[10] Burns further modified Dieterle's method for the identification of intestinal spirochetes.[11] In the late 1980s, microwave oven variations, offering reduced staining times along with cleaner and clearer results for staining spirochetes, entered the literature.[12-15] Elias and Bosma[16] and especially Garvey et al[17-19] have worked extensively with modifications of the original Steiner method.

The silver impregnation procedures for bacteria, like those mentioned, blacken all organisms nonselectively and are excellent for demonstrating the thin, weakly gram-negative spirochetes. All of these procedures depend on the precipitation, or accretion, of silver ions onto the argyrophilic surface of the bacterial cell wall, leaving the tissue cells only slightly colored.[20] Regardless of the method, the development of this impregnated clear silver salt to a visible, black metallic form in a "physical" reducing solution is the critical part of this technique. In a brilliant article published in 2002, Kiernan[21] eloquently described the exact mechanisms involved in silver staining of spirochetes in paraffin sections of formaldehyde-fixed specimens: "This is a simple method; only two of its steps are actively involved in staining the bacteria...the first stage of the procedure involves the formation of submicroscopic clusters ('nuclei') of silver atoms in the bacteria. In the second step, these nuclei catalyze local reduction of more silver ions by a reducing agent until enough colloidal metal has been deposited to display the organisms as black objects of characteristic form."

As has been described, the literature contains many modifications and helpful hints about how to achieve clearly delineated spirochetes, with minimal background and connective tissue staining. However, anyone who has worked with and performed these techniques is familiar with just how capricious they can be. A balance must be achieved between underdevelopment, which results in pale-staining, thin organisms against a pale or clear background, and overdevelopment, which results in thick, black organisms against a dark yellow-brown background. To the naked eye, an underdeveloped section is pale yellow, and an overdeveloped section is dark golden brown. Automated special staining platforms utilizing standardized reagents, conditions, and staining times have made these methods more reproducible.

Perhaps one of the simplest and most reproducible methods for staining spirochetes manually in tissue sections is the "revised" modified Steiner method described by Garvey et al.[18] This method uses a very dilute solution of uranyl nitrate (0.1%) as a pretreatment to block silver uptake in nerve fibers that can mimic organisms. A very dilute silver nitrate solution (0.1%), heated to precisely 70°C, is used for impregnation, which makes the technique very affordable. The reducing solution, consisting of gum mastic, hydroquinone, and a small amount of silver, is easy to make and effective.

To improve safety and address the potential radioactive hazard involved in its use, some authors have recommended replacing the uranyl nitrate pretreatment solution with lead nitrate,[22] zinc-formalin,[23] or phosphotungstic acid.[24] Both lead nitrate and zinc-formalin have proved to be somewhat effective for demonstrating spirochetes, but phosphotungstic acid has not. The Warthin Starry method (and some of its modifications) is a popular alternative technique because neither uranyl nitrate nor any pretreatment reagent is required for staining most bacteria. However, when staining for spirochetes, it is clear that without some form of pretreatment, they will stain poorly or not at all.[25]

Reduction of nonspecific background staining, perhaps the most common problem, has been the focus of several authors, who have modified existing methods by improving the impregnation of the spirochetes themselves using various pretreatments. Others have suggested that lowering the concentrations of the various chemicals used in the procedure is effective in preventing staining of connective tissue and/or nuclei. Garvey et al have suggested that preheating, along with the concentration of the silver solution used for impregnation, the amount of silver and hydroquinone in the reducing solution, and the staining temperature are all critical factors in obtaining reduced nonspecific background staining.[18]

Formalin pigment and calcium salts present in silver-stained sections can cause the sections to appear dirty and may even be confused with bacterial organisms. These deposits may be removed by treating sections with 10% phenol/10% HCl/absolute ethanol for 10 minutes, followed by a 20% formic acid solution for 10 minutes.[19] Formalin pigment and calcium salts can also be removed using 1% amylase at 60°C for 1 to 2 hours.[16]

Dirty glassware, including the slides that carry the sections, can reduce silver and cause nonspecific background staining. The worst form of contaminant is metallic silver remaining in Coplin jars from earlier use. All glassware, including reagent bottles, should be cleaned with nitric acid and rinsed with distilled or deionized water. If chloride ions are present in any of the solutions (eg, from tap water), silver chloride forms and is partly reduced to silver by the action of light.[21] Gelatin and gum mastic may contain impurities and cause nonspecific reduction of silver and increased nonspecific staining. These components should be chemical grade and obtained from a reliable chemical vendor. Clean glassware, pure reagents, and avoidance of contamination have long been recognized as essential for the success of traditional silver-staining techniques and their modern variants.

In practice, with any silver method for spirochetes, it is advisable to process at least three sections plus a positive control for each and to try three different developing times.[1] If only one section is available and nonspecific deposition of silver occurs, it may be worth trying to remove it with brief rinses in a 0.5% potassium ferricyanide solution.[26] A comparison of common silver methods used for staining spirochetes along with their published modifications is found in Table 8.2

Controls
It is essential to understand that, when performing these techniques, proper control material must be used. Spirochetes range in size from 0.075 to 0.200 μm in width and 6 to 25 μm in length and are considerably smaller and thinner than most other bacteria. Therefore, any method used for their demonstration must be optimized using tissues known to contain spirochetes. If other bacteria are used, such as *Helicobacter pylori*, which can be up to 5 times the width of typical spirochetes, the accretion of the reduced silver on these bacteria causes them to appear larger and considerably easier to demonstrate. To assure detection, and as a "rigorous test" of the staining protocol and method sensitivity, spirochete control material is required.

What Should Be Seen in a Good Stain for Spirochetes
Regardless of the method used, spirochetes should be distinctly black, spiral-shaped, rodlike organisms of variable length against a yellowish-tan to light brown background. The observer must be aware that all spirochete methods will stain calcium salts, formalin pigment, and melanin pigment very distinctly. These substances may be the cause of unwanted background staining but are unavoidable unless removed before the silver impregnation step. Examples of good spirochete stains are seen in Figures 8.1 through 8.4.

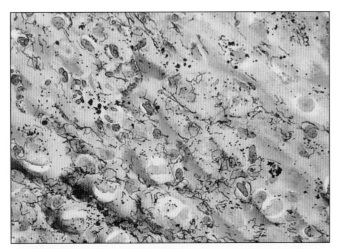

Figure 8.1. Numerous *Treponema palladium* organisms are present in this section of skin stained with the modified Steiner technique. The coarse black substance in the background is melanin pigment.

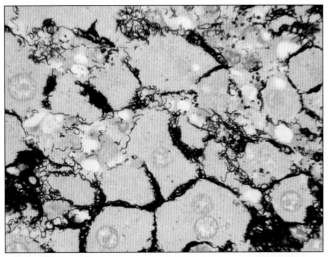

Figure 8.2. In this section of liver stained with the Warthin-Starry method, the sinusoids are distended by numerous *Leptospira*.

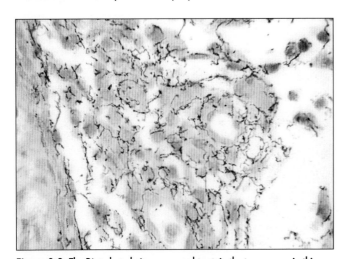

Figure 8.3. The Dieterle technique was used to stain the treponemes in this section of rat testis.

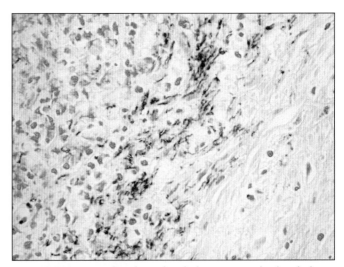

Figure 8.4. An immunohistochemical method using a monoclonal antibody was used to stain the spirochetes present in the wall of the umbilical cord in this case of congenital syphilis. Distinct helical morphology is often obscured when using immunohistochemistry.

Problems Encountered With Stains for Spirochetes

PROBLEM: Understained or Unstained Organisms

APPEARANCE: Spirochetes in known positive control sections are not seen or are only minimally stained and the background is colorless or very light yellow (Figures 8.5 and 8.6).

CAUSES:

- Sections were not properly exposed or not exposed at all to a pretreatment solution (ie, 0.1% to 1.0% aqueous uranyl nitrate).
- Sections were not immersed long enough in silver impregnation solution.
- Silver impregnation solution was not adequately heated.
- Tissue sections were underexposed to developing solutions.
- Developing solution was improperly made.

SOLUTIONS:

- Staining for spirochetes requires a pretreatment step; use according to protocol.
- Best results are achieved if the silver solution is heated to between 60° and 70°C. Be careful if using microwave heating; water bath heating is highly reliable and recommended if performing the technique manually.

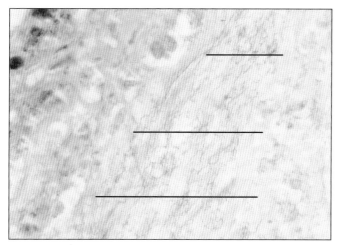

Figure 8.5. The numerous organisms are badly understained and the background is very light as a result of removing the section from the developing solution before adequate contrast was obtained. Organisms, which should be distinctly black, are present above and below each of the three horizontal lines.

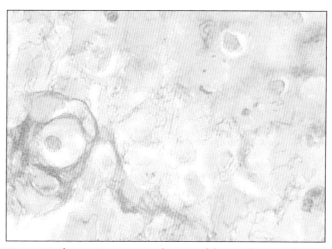

Figure 8.6. The organisms present in the center of this spirochete control section are very understained. The section was immersed in silver nitrate solution that was not adequately heated and was subsequently removed too soon from the developer, resulting in lack of contrast.

- Increase time in the developing solution; assure that it is correctly preheated. Check results microscopically before coverslipping.
- Assure that the developing solution is precisely made according to directions using fresh reagents.

COMMENTS: Underdeveloped stains can be returned to the developing solution to deepen the color of the organisms and provide better contrast. Results are best when fresh solutions are used throughout this staining procedure.

PROBLEM: Nonspecific Background Staining; Silver Precipitate; Undesirable Tissue Structures Stained Too Darkly; Reduced Contrast, Making Detection of Organisms Difficult

APPEARANCE: Spirochetes are stained, but detection is compromised or totally obscured because of nonspecific brown-black staining of nuclei, cellular debris, connective tissue fibers, peripheral nerve fibers, melanin pigment, calcium salts, and/or formalin pigment (Figures 8.7 through 8.10).

CAUSES:

- The silver impregnation solution is too hot.
- Tissue sections are overexposed to developing solutions.
- The developing solution contains too much hydroquinone or silver nitrate.
- Silver nitrate solutions are not freshly made.

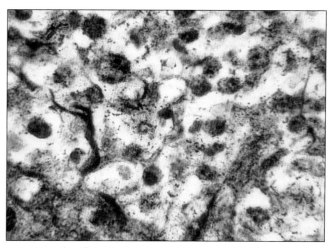

Figure 8.7. The cells in this control section are covered with silver precipitate as a result of overheating the silver solution during impregnation. It appears that some helical structures may be stained, but it is difficult to discern the difference between actual bacteria and granular background staining.

SOLUTIONS:

- Preheat silver impregnation solutions; check temperature and stir slides into both silver and developer and agitate. Use of a water bath is recommended.
- Monitor color development of sections by checking slides at regular intervals (eg, 3, 6, 9, and 12 minutes).
- Use multiple sections of the same block, each with matched controls, and remove them from developer at different times.

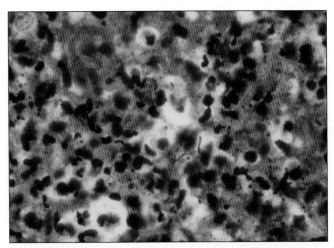

Figure 8.8. This spirochete control section was overdeveloped. The dark nuclei and cell cytoplasm decrease the contrast, making identification of organisms difficult. Generally, this appearance is caused by improper formulation of, or overexposure to, the reducing solution, or both.

- Assure that the developing solution is properly made according to exact specifications of the technique being used.
- Use freshly prepared reagents and "clean" technique for each step of the protocol.

COMMENTS: Perhaps the most common type of problem associated with silver impregnation techniques for spirochetes is the one described above. An unduly high temperature of silver nitrate is a common cause of precipitate and high background, and darkly stained fibrin, reticulin, or elastin fibers can be confused with spirochetes.[19] However, proper formulation and use of the reducing solution can alleviate many problems. It has been demonstrated that the concentrations of hydroquinone and silver in the developing solution are critical to avoid background staining. Hydroquinone, at a concentration above or below 0.625%, causes improper development or staining of the spirochetes. Freshly prepared silver at a concentration above 0.01% causes nuclei to stain. Increasing the amount of silver in the reducing solution causes the development to proceed at a faster rate but also causes the connective tissue and the background to stain more intensely.[18] Strict attention to detail and accurate formulation of the reducing solution is essential in achieving optimal contrast between the organisms and the background. Monitoring of development times and using multiple sections and slides, as described, cannot be overemphasized; however, some tissue components can be expected to stain darkly even when the technique is correctly performed. These components include melanin; the cytoplasmic granules of

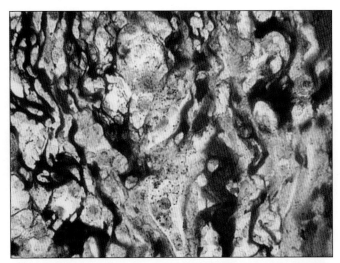

Figure 8.9. Connective tissue fibers are darkened in this section stained with the Warthin-Starry method. Adding excessive silver nitrate to the developing solution will cause collagen and reticulin fibers to stain intensely. In addition, the silver impregnation solution may have been overheated, because silver precipitate is present.

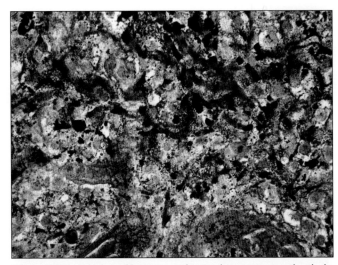

Figure 8.10. Multiple problems are evident in this section stained with the Steiner technique. Silver precipitate is present throughout the background, formalin pigment is present, and the connective tissue fibers and some nuclei are stained. Contrast is totally compromised, making accurate identification of spirochetes difficult.

some endocrine cells, which contain reducing substances; and chromatin within some cell nuclei. Overstained sections can be lightened or destained, but the solution used affects the staining of the spirochetes as well as the background. Optimal results are obtained only by strict attention to detail, careful handling, and practice.

References

1. Bancroft JD, Stevens A. *Theory and Practice of Histological Techniques.* 3rd ed. Edinburgh, UK: Churchill Livingstone; 1990: 187-189.

2. Elias JM. Infectious organisms: meeting the new challenge in surgical pathology. *J Histotechnol.* 1995;18:177-178.

3. Cartun RW. Use of immunohistochemistry in the surgical pathology laboratory for the diagnosis of infectious diseases. *Pathol Case Rev.* 1999;4:260-265.

4. Levaditi C. Sur la coloration de Spirochaete pallida Schaudinn dans les coupes. *Comptes rendus des seances de la societe de biologie et de ses flliales.* 1905;59(2):326.

5. Warthin AS, Starry AC. A more rapid and improved method for demonstrating spirochetes in tissue. *Am J Syph Gonorr Ven Dis.* 1920;4:97-102.

6. Dieterle RR. Method for demonstration of Spirochaeta pallida in single microscopic sections. *Arch Neurol Psychiatr.* 1927;18:73-80.

7. Kerr DA. Improved Warthin-Starry method of staining spirochetes in tissue sections. *Am J Clin Pathol.* 1938;8:63-67.

8. Faulkner RR, Lillie RD. A buffer modification of the Warthin-Starry silver method for spirochetes in single paraffin sections. *Stain Technol.* 1945;20(3):8l-82.

9. Steiner G, Steiner U. New simple silver stain for demonstration of bacteria, spirochetes, and fungi in sections from paraffin embedded tissue blocks. *J Lab Clin Med.* 1944;29:868-871.

10. Van Orden AE, Greer PW. Modification of Dieterle spirochete stain. *J Histotechnol.* 1977;1:51-53.

11. Burns A. Staining intestinal spirochetes. *Med Lab Sci.* 1982;39:75-77.

12. Vail KF. The Warthin-Starry impregnation technique with the microwave oven. *HistoLogic.* 1987;17:235-236.

13. Churukian C. A Warthin-Starry method for spirochetes and bacteria using a microwave oven. *J Histotechnol.* 1988;13:149-151.

14. Swisher LS. Modified Steiner procedure for microwave staining of spirochetes and nonfilamentous bacteria. *J Histotechnol.* 1987;10:241-243.

15. Churukian C, Garvey W. Microwave Steiner method for spirochetes and bacteria. *J Histotechnol.* 1990;13:45-47.

16. Elias EA, Bosma R. Silver staining for microorganisms in tissue sections of paraffin and plastic embedded material. *Cell Mol Biol.* 1987;33(6):711-723.

17. Garvey W, Fathi A, Bigelow F. Modified Steiner for the demonstration of spirochetes. *J Histotechnol.* 1985;8:5-17.

18. Garvey W, Fathi A, Bigelow F, Wynnchuk M. Revised modified Steiner to enhance visibility of spirochetes. *J Histotechnol.* 1995;18:57-60.

19. Garvey F. Silver impregnation techniques to identify spirochetes and other bacteria. *J Histotechnol.* 1996;19:203-209.

20. Winn WC. Current concepts in pathologic diagnosis. *J Histotechnol.* 1995;18:241-246.

21. Kiernan JA. Silver staining for spirochetes in tissues: rationale, difficulties, and troubleshooting. *Lab Med.* 2002;33:705-708.

22. Elias JM, Green C. Modified Steiner method for the demonstration of spirochetes in tissue. *Am J Clin Pathol.* 1979;71:109-111.

23. Margeson LS, Chapman CM. Use of zinc formalin as a sensitizer in silver stains for spirochetes. *J Histotechnol.* 1996;19:135-138.

24. Buesa, RJ. Phosphotungstic acid eliminates uranyl nitrate as a sensitizer before the silver impregnation of Helicobacter pylori. *J Histotechnol.* 2001;24:113-116.

25. Churukian C. A Warthin-Starry method for spirochetes and bacteria using a microwave oven. *J Histotechnol.* 1988;13:149-151.

26. Carson FL. *Histotechnology: A Self-Instructional Text.* 2nd ed. Chicago, IL: American Society of Clinical Pathologists; 1997: 196-197.

Fungi

Robert L. Lott

Although fungi are ubiquitous in nature, they are primarily involved in the degradation of organic waste material; very few fungi cause human disease. Humans have a high level of innate immunity to fungi, and most of the infections they cause are mild and self-limiting. Among the most common fungal infections in humans are the superficial or cutaneous mycoses, such as those caused by *Microsporum* and *Trichophyton*. The systemic mycoses, such as those caused by *Blastomyces*, *Coccidioides*, and *Histoplasma*, originate primarily in the lungs but can spread to many organ systems. These organisms are inherently virulent and can cause life-threatening infections. The opportunistic fungi, such as *Candida*, *Cryptococcus*, and *Aspergillus*, are generally considered nonpathogenic and can be found in normal respiratory secretions; increasingly, however, they cause disseminated infections in immunocompromised and immunosuppressed individuals.[1]

Some fungi may elicit host tissue reactions ranging from exudative to granulomatous; other fungi produce little cellular response.[2] Microscopically, fungal organisms may appear as a vegetative growth with filamentous hyphae, a tubular form that may exhibit branching. Reproductive forms may appear to be forming buds. Asexual yeast forms appear as rounded spores that may or may not be apparent in a hematoxylin-and-eosin (H&E)–stained slide. Most fungi can be seen with the H&E stain, appearing variably, but usually weakly, basophilic (Figure 9.1). In general, the fungal wall has a low affinity for hematoxylin—hence the need for special staining techniques that can make the organisms more readily apparent.

Special staining methods take advantage of the fact that the walls of fungal organisms are rich in complex carbohydrates (polysaccharides). These carbohydrates are oxidized to form reactive aldehyde groups, which can then be detected with a silver solution (Gomori methenamine silver [GMS] stain) or by the Schiff reaction (periodic acid–Schiff [PAS] or Gridley). Metachromatic dye solutions may also be of value in circumstances where a rapid stain is desired.[3]

Grocott's modification of the GMS technique[4] or one of its rapid variants remain the most popular method for

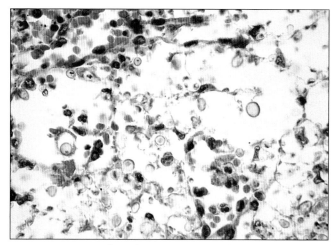

Figure 9.1. Hematoxylin and eosin (H&E) stain of fungus control section. The walls of the fungal spores are weakly basophilic and lightly stained with hematoxylin.

identifying fungi in tissue sections. Fungi are visualized by the action of the aldehyde groups created after oxidation of fungal wall components. These newly formed aldehydes have the ability to both bind the clear silver nitrate and reduce it to a visible metallic form. Despite the challenges and idiosyncrasies of silver impregnation techniques, the properly performed GMS stain offers optimal staining sensitivity and contrast, particularly for smaller organisms, such as *Pneumocystis laroveci* (formerly *P carinii*), that may otherwise be masked in a mucinous, inflammatory exudate typically caused by this organism. It is the best method for the detection of fungi in tissue sections, particularly when they are present in small numbers. The black-staining fungi stand out prominently against a clear background.

In most instances, the GMS procedures will stain old and nonviable organisms, which are often not detected with the PAS and Gridley procedures. When properly performed, the GMS method usually eliminates nonspecific background staining of normal tissue components and necrotic debris, whereas the PAS and Gridley procedures do not. The GMS stain is also more sensitive because it demonstrates certain nonfungal pathogens, such as *Actinomyces* and *Nocardia* species, *Mycobacterium* species, nonfilamentous bacteria with polysaccharide capsules, certain algal cells (eg, *Prototheca* and *Chlorella*), the spores of certain microsporidia, and the cytoplasmic granular inclusion bodies of cytomegalovirus. Such an all-purpose, low-specificity stain is extremely helpful for rapid screening of specimens from patients with acquired immune deficiency syndrome (AIDS), who are often infected by multiple pathogens.[5]

In the GMS stain, oxidation with chromic acid will reduce the staining of background tissue structures, such as reticulin, collagen, and basement membranes. These connective tissue fibers contain a much smaller percentage of carbohydrate than do fungal walls. Chromic acid, a strong oxidant, acts to convert the carbohydrate content of these fibers to aldehydes, but, because they are so few in number, they are oxidized past the aldehyde stage to form carboxyl groups that will not react. These breakdown products do not bind silver because they are much weaker reducing agents than are aldehyde groups.[6] Therefore, background staining is prevented in connective tissue fibers by oxidizing their native carbohydrate content "past the point" of their ability to bind the silver solution. Conversely, inadequate oxidation of these structures causes the carbohydrate component in mucin, reticulin fibers, collagen, and basement membranes to stain. This background staining can mask the fungal organisms if it is severe enough or if fungal organisms are sparse.

Typically, the impregnation step is carried out with a strongly alkaline, aqueous solution of silver hexamethamine (methenamine); however, in 1986, Churukian et al introduced a silver staining solution for fungi that does not use methenamine at all.[7] It uses a very dilute, alkaline, ammoniacal silver solution prepared much like the ammoniacal silver used when staining for reticulin. One advantage of this formulation appears to be its stability when heated. It can be vigorously heated in a microwave oven, speeding up the staining reaction, and it will not precipitate, break down, or produce random silver deposits on the glass side ("mirroring") below temperatures of 80° to 85°C. Tome et al also preferred ammoniacal silver and stated, "this new method yields more consistent results in fungal staining without background staining, and is considered superior to Grocott's methenamine method with regard to its simplicity and reproducibility."[8]

When GMS staining is performed manually, care must be taken not to overstain with the working silver solution. Overstaining occurs typically when tissue sections are left too long in the working silver solution or when the solution is too warm (above 65°C). When sections are overstained, basement membranes of capillaries and venules become darkened and can mimic fungal

hyphae, particularly if the vessels are branched and empty. Overstained erythrocytes and naked nuclei can mimic yeasts. Reticulin and elastic fibers can be mistaken for filamentous bacteria. Calcific bodies, which often look like yeast cells, are dissolved by the chromic acid used in the GMS and Gridley procedures and are therefore unstained; however, they do stain with H&E and the PAS reaction.[9] It is interesting to note that this type of overstaining occurs *even when sections have been properly oxidized* with chromic acid to suppress nonspecific staining. This phenomenon reinforces the need for microscopic determination of the staining end point as well as standardization of all variables within the procedure.

The blackened silver end product against a clear light background lends itself to a variety of counterstains. Specific nuclear stains, such as neutral red or methylene blue, or a variety of cytoplasmic stains, such as light green, safranin O, or metanil yellow, may be used. Using an H&E counterstain with the GMS procedure allows simultaneous evaluation of both fungal morphology and the inflammatory response. Tissue sections stained using this modification are ideal for teaching and photomicrography.[10]

The PAS reaction is often performed in place of the GMS stain to detect fungi, especially in dermatologic specimens. In the PAS reaction, the polysaccharides in the fungal wall are converted to aldehyde groups with periodic acid. The newly formed aldehydes bind the Schiff reagent, and subsequent washing with water "recolorizes" the Schiff reagent, yielding a fuchsia-pink color. According to Della Speranza, chromic acid should be used as the oxidizer for the demonstration of fungal walls, whereas weaker oxidizers such as periodic acid should be used only for the demonstration of basement membranes and reticulin fibers.[11] The use of periodic acid in the PAS procedure may lead to the staining of undesirable tissue elements. Because periodic acid will not oxidize carbohydrate components past the aldehyde stage, tissue structures that contain even small amounts of carbohydrate, such as reticulin, collagen, and basement membranes, are stained. Which method (GMS vs PAS) is utilized to demonstrate fungal organisms is often a matter of preference; however, *Histoplasma capsulatum* and *Pneumocystis laroveci* are not adequately demonstrated by the PAS reaction,[12] whereas the GMS method will stain both of the above, as well as dead and viable fungal organisms.

Some fungi, such as *Cryptococcus neoformans*, are surrounded by a thick mucoid capsule. A mucicarmine, Alcian blue, or colloidal iron stain may be a useful aid in identifying these encapsulated yeasts (Figure 9.2); however, they are not specific for this particular fungus. *Blastomyces* and *Rhinosporidium* may also be stained with the mucin stains.

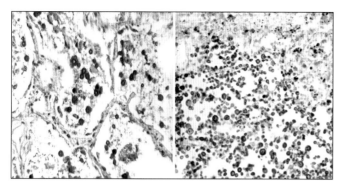

Figure 9.2. Known *Cryptococcus* control sections stained with mucicarmine (left) and colloidal iron (right).

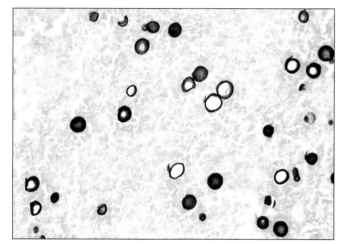

Figure 9.3. A well-stained Gomori methenamine silver (GMS) control section of lung demonstrating the thick fungal walls of *Blastomyces dermatitidis* against a clean, light green background.

Controls

Tissues known to contain fungal organisms must be used as the positive control for these techniques. Control sections that contain fungal spores and hyphae are optimal for PAS stains. When staining for *Pneumocystis jaroveci*, tissues known to contain this organism should be included in the control because of the delicate nature of its cell wall, thereby allowing for proper microscopic determination of the staining end point.

What Should Be Seen in a Good Stain for Fungi

Regardless of the method used, fungi should be distinct and well delineated. With the GMS stain, fungal walls should appear black, and the internal structure of the organism should be observable against a good background counterstain (Figures 9.3, 9.4, and 9.5) A well-stained GMS slide should be essentially free of nonspecific silver staining, but this is not so with a PAS stain for fungus. If periodic acid is used as the oxidizer in this method, collagen, reticulin, and basement membranes will be stained (Figure 9.6). If chromic acid is substituted

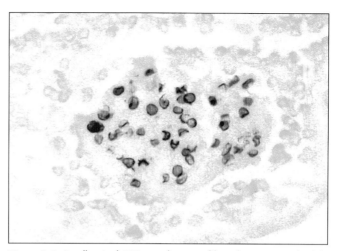

Figure 9.4. A well-stained GMS control section of lung demonstrating the delicate walls of *Pneumocystis laroveci* against a clean, light green background.

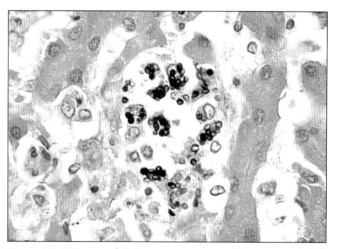

Figure 9.5. GMS stain with H&E counterstain is an excellent way to study both the fungal infection and the associated cellular response.

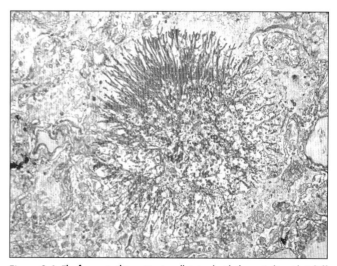

Figure 9.6. The fungus in this section is well stained with the periodic acid–Schiff (PAS) reaction. This section of lung is counterstained with light green. Note that the collagen and alveolar cell walls are lightly stained with this technique.

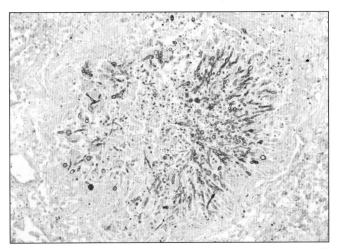

Figure 9.7. The fungus in this section is well stained with the chromic acid–Schiff reaction. No background connective tissue structures are stained.

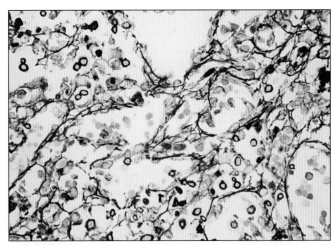

Figure 9.8. The thick-walled *Cryptococcus neoformans* microorganisms in this section are well stained; however, inadequate oxidation has caused the connective tissue fibers in the alveolar septa to stain also.

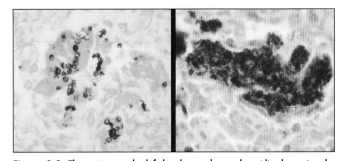

Figure 9.9. The section on the left has been adequately oxidized, causing the mucinous background to be suppressed. The contrast between the *Pneumocystis* organisms and the background is excellent. The section on the right has not been properly oxidized and contrast is absent.

as the oxidizing agent, it is possible to suppress these undesirable elements so that the fungi appear distinct[11] (Figure 9.7).

Problems Encountered With Silver Stains for Fungi

PROBLEM: Inadequate Oxidation; Occurrence of Nonspecific Staining in Tissue Elements Other Than Fungi

APPEARANCE: Fungi are stained, but other tissue structures, such as mucin, collagen, reticulin fibers, basement membranes, and/or nuclei, are also stained (Figure 9.8).

CAUSES:

- The chromic acid oxidizing solution may be exhausted or old.
- Oxidation time is inadequate.
- The strength of the oxidizer solution may be incorrect.
- A weak oxidizer like periodic acid will contribute to nonspecific staining. Reducing sites are not quenched on reticulin fibers and basement membranes, thus causing silver ions to bind. Periodic acid should not be substituted for chromic acid in the GMS method because it results in increased background staining and is less effective in identifying some organisms, such as *Histoplasma capsulatum*.[12]

SOLUTIONS:

- Regularly replace or refresh the chromic acid solution used for oxidation, especially if the solution color changes in any way.
- Validate oxidation times using chromic acid only by continually experimenting with known positive controls.
- Although hardly practical, some authors recommend carrying out the stain in the dark to prevent the reducing action of ambient light on the silver impregnation solution.

COMMENTS: The importance of proper oxidation cannot be overemphasized. When a slide is properly oxidized and stained using the GMS method for fungus, little else will stain other than the fungal organisms contained in the section (see Figure 9.9).

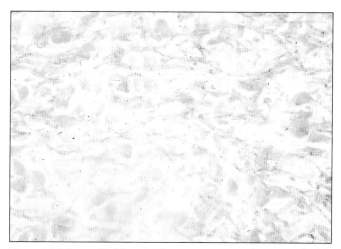

Figure 9.10. Distinct black fungal walls are not apparent in this section. The slide was removed from the working silver solution before adequate silver impregnation occurred, resulting in very light, inadequate staining

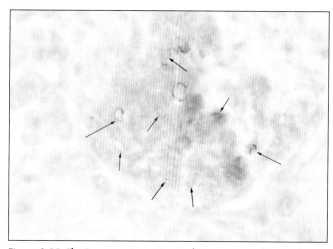

Figure 9.11. The *Pneumocystis* organisms in this section are understained. Some are only partially stained, and some are not stained at all. Arrows indicate the location of possible organisms.

PROBLEM: Understaining of Fungal Organisms

APPEARANCE: Organisms are very faintly stained or only partially stained and lack a clearly delineated black cell wall. These organisms often appear light brown or may be partially or completely unstained (Figures 9.10, 9.11, and 9.12).

CAUSES:

- Oxidation is inadequate to expose all potential reducing sites in the fungal wall.

- Tissues are not exposed to the working silver solution for a sufficient time.

- Working silver solution is not adequately heated.

SOLUTIONS:

- Validate oxidation times using chromic acid *only* by continually experimenting with known positive controls.

- Ideally, all reducing sites will be saturated with silver ions, but this reaction is both time and temperature dependent. Staining end point must be determined microscopically to ensure optimal staining.

COMMENTS: It is important to understand that understaining of fungal organisms can easily lead to a misdiagnosis that has important clinical implications for the patient. *Histoplasma* or *Pneumocystis*, for example, may cause extensive disease, although often only a few organisms may be present. If the tissue is inadequately stained, the patient may receive a false-negative diagnosis and go untreated.

Figure 9.12. This section contains *Candida albicans* that is moderately understained. Some fungal cell walls are well defined and internal structure is evident, while others are only faintly stained.

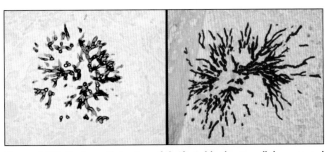

Figure 9.13. The internal structure of the fungal hyphae is well demonstrated in the section on the left. The section on the right has been slightly overstained, with no apparent internal structure.

PROBLEM: Overstaining of Fungal Organisms

APPEARANCE: Organisms present are completely blackened to the point that no internal structure, such as hyphal septae, within the organism is observed microscopically (Figure 9.13). Typically, when sections are left in the silver solution too long, reticular fibers, red blood cells, and other tissue structures may be stained non-specifically[13] (Figures 9.14 and 9.15).

CAUSES:

• The working methenamine silver solution is over-heated to temperatures above 62° to 65°C.

• Sections are left too long in the warm, working silver solution.

SOLUTIONS:

• Avoid heating the silver impregnation solution above 62°C because this may contribute to the breakdown of the staining solution.

• The working silver solution should be allowed to reach 60° to 62°C before the slides are inserted. Heating the solution in a Coplin jar in a water bath is more efficient than heating in a convection oven.

• Microwave heating must be worked out in advance to avoid overheating. It is often most efficient to gently warm the working silver solution in the microwave and transfer to a water bath to avoid overheating.

COMMENTS: Overstaining may mask the presence of fungal organisms and is to be avoided. Fibrin strands may stain black, particularly in overincubated sections, but are rarely confused with fungal hyphae, the latter being much thicker. Overstaining of tissue sections is often due to overexposure to the working methenamine silver solution even when proper oxidation has been carried out. Tissue sections are often left in the solution for too long, or the solution is overheated. Microscopic determination of the end point is key to successful staining. It is very important that the internal structure of the

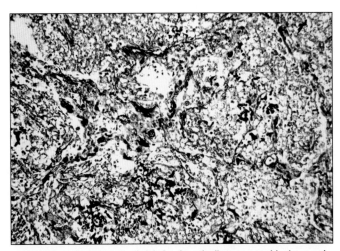

Figure 9.14. This GMS-stained slide has been badly overstained by leaving the section in the working silver solution too long. Fungal organisms are stained, but contrast is compromised, with essentially all structures in the background labeled nonspecifically with silver.

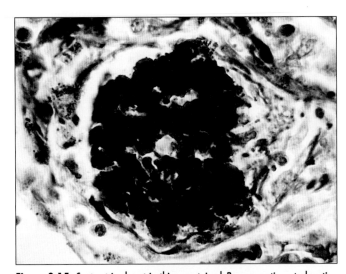

Figure 9.15. Contrast is absent in this overstained *Pneumocystis* control section as a result of overheating of the working silver solution. Cell nuclei, mucin, and connective tissue are stained nonspecifically.

organisms be visualized. Such detail is seen best in a slightly underincubated section.

PROBLEM: Random Deposition of Silver Onto the Glass Slide ("Mirroring") or the Staining Vessel

APPEARANCE: Metallic silver is deposited nonspecifically over large areas of the front and back of the glass slide. The silver solution deposits a fine, brown-black, granular precipitate over the section and the glass portion of the slide (Figures 9.16 and 9.17). Microscopically, this type of precipitate is usually not in the same plane as the tissue.

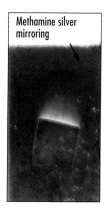

Figure 9.16. The methenamine silver solution was overheated, causing it to break down and randomly deposit silver particles (or "mirror") onto the glass slide.

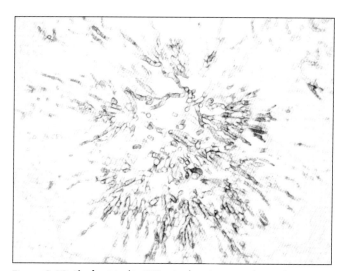

Figure 9.18. The fungi in this GMS-stained section are undertoned, appearing brown rather than a distinct black color. No counterstain is present.

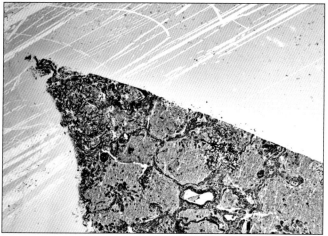

Figure 9.17. The result of overheating the methenamine silver solution is apparent in this section. In addition to the "mirroring," the section shows non-specific staining.

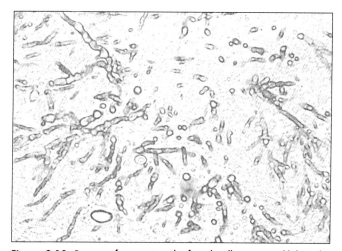

Figure 9.19. Because of overtoning, the fungal walls appear reddish in this GMS-stained section, with no counterstain.

CAUSES:

- Working methenamine silver has been overheated during the impregnation step.

- Glassware or plastic Coplin jar is contaminated with reagents from previous use.

SOLUTIONS:

- Avoid heating the silver impregnation solution above 60° to 62°C both before and during its use.

- Use ammoniacal silver for impregnation step.

- Use of acid-cleaned glassware is recommended.

COMMENTS: Mirroring of metallic silver onto the slide is a clear sign that the working methenamine silver solution has been overheated either before or during its use. Methodology should be employed and validated in the laboratory so that the silver solution is properly heated (to about 60°C) to assure impregnation, but not overheated, contributing to the breakdown of the solution. Ammoniacal silver solutions are much more stable when vigorously heated (ie, using microwave) and will not

break down or mirror the slides under normal staining conditions. In addition, acid-cleaned glassware should always be used for these staining techniques; this cleaning method is intended to remove soap, stain residues, and other chemical remnants from the staining vessel that may react with the impregnation solution. Slides should be transferred into and out of the impregnation solution with nonmetallic forceps.

PROBLEM: Undertoning or Overtoning of Stained Organisms

APPEARANCE: If undertoned, stained fungal structures appear a golden-brown or yellow (Figure 9.18) instead of black; if overtoned, they take on a reddish hue (Figure 9.19).

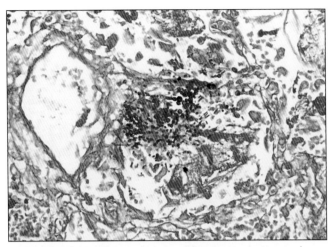

Figure 9.20. The small fungi in the center of this PAS-stained section are demonstrated; however, contrast is compromised by the use of periodic acid as the oxidizing solution, which also stains the connective tissue in the background.

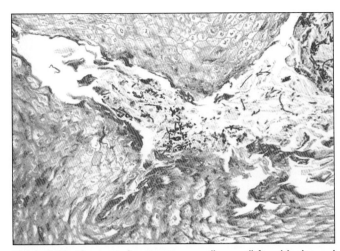

Figure 9.21. Glycogen in keratinocytes, as well as small fungal hyphae and spores, is demonstrated in this PAS-stained section, which is counterstained with hematoxylin.

CAUSES:

- Underexposure to the gold chloride will stain the organisms light- to golden-brown or yellow.

- Overexposure to the gold chloride solution will produce a reddish hue.

SOLUTIONS:

- To prevent undertoning, increase the exposure time to gold chloride or use a fresh gold chloride solution.

- To prevent overtoning, reduce the time of exposure or reduce the strength of the gold chloride.

COMMENTS: Correctly stained fungal structures typically should appear black under the microscope. This color is achieved by exposing silver deposits to a gold chloride solution, where the gold particles compete for and add to the deposited silver particles, a procedure referred to as *toning*. Prolonged toning creates a reddish hue of the silver-stained structures. Silver deposits that fail to take on the desired black coloration are said to be undertoned (ie, insufficiently toned). Undertoning may occur if sections are exposed to gold chloride for an insufficient period of time, but more commonly it occurs because the gold chloride solution is exhausted. This outcome may be remedied by increasing the section's exposure to gold chloride or by using a fresh gold chloride solution for toning.

Problems Encountered With Periodic Acid-Schiff Stains for Fungi

PROBLEM: Background Staining and Lack of Contrast

APPEARANCE: Along with the specific staining of fungal organisms, the PAS reaction stains the native carbohydrate content of tissue elements (eg, glycogen, collagen, basement membranes, and mucin) a pink-red color. The result is that fungi can be difficult to visualize, and the contrast between the organisms and the background is reduced.

CAUSES:

- Use of a weak oxidizing solution, such as periodic acid, can cause this artifact. Periodic acid will not oxidize the native carbohydrate-containing background elements past the aldehyde stage, thus allowing these elements, along with the carbohydrate-rich fungal walls, to react with the Schiff reagent (Figures 9.20 and 9.21).

- Old, depleted, or decomposing Schiff reagent can cause this problem.

SOLUTIONS:

- Use a strong oxidizer. Chromic acid is recommended when performing the PAS reaction for staining fungus (Figure 9.22).

- Use fresh Schiff reagent.

COMMENTS: The normal oxidizing reagent used in the PAS reaction, periodic acid, should be replaced with chromic acid when staining for microorganisms is performed. Chromic acid is capable of oxidizing the native carbohydrate content (typically low) in collagen, base-

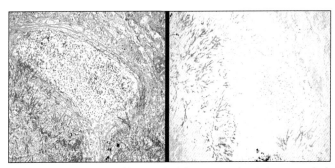

Figure 9.22. The section of lung on the left was stained with the PAS method, using periodic acid as the oxidizer. The same section on the right was stained with a chromic acid–Schiff (CAS) technique. Fungi are demonstrated in both sections; however, staining of the background is suppressed with the CAS method.

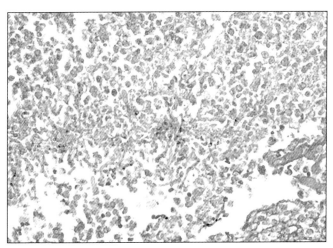

Figure 9.23. In this PAS-stained section, fungi are only faintly stained because a depleted Schiff reagent was used.

ment membranes, and mucin "past" the aldehyde stage, making the resulting moieties unavailable to bind the Schiff reagent. Thus, background interference from these tissue structures is virtually eliminated. Fungal walls are very rich in complex carbohydrate. The short exposure to chromic acid affects them to some degree, but enough of their content is preserved to allow staining with the Schiff reagent.

PROBLEM: Weak Staining or No Staining of Fungal Elements in Control Sections

APPEARANCE: Light pink, nonspecific background staining occurs across the entire section. Fungi stained with the PAS reaction do not exhibit the bright red-magenta color associated with Schiff reagent. Fungal elements are a dull red and only faintly stained or not stained at all (Figure 9.23).

CAUSES:
- Oxidizer is exhausted, old, or diluted (chromic acid or periodic acid).
- Old, depleted, or decomposing Schiff reagent is used.

SOLUTIONS:
- Use fresh oxidizer. Chromic acid is recommended when performing the PAS reaction for staining fungus.
- Use fresh Schiff reagent.

COMMENTS: The use of a freshly prepared oxidizing solution and fresh Schiff reagent will virtually guarantee successful staining. Pink background staining may be due to the decomposition of the Schiff reagent, which is probably the result of extensive use, aging, carryover of periodate, contamination or dilution by water, or thermal decomposition during microwave-accelerated stain-

ing. Schiff reagent that has turned pink after being heated in a microwave can often be restored to its clear appearance by returning the solution to the refrigerator for a period of time.

References

1. Bancroft J, Stevens A. *Theory and Practice of Histological Techniques.* 2nd ed. New York, NY: Churchill Livingstone; 1982: 278-296.

2. Bancroft J, Gamble M. *Theory and Practice of Histological Techniques.* 5th ed. New York, NY: Churchill Livingstone; 2002: 335-336.

3. Gosey L, Howard R, Witebsky F, et al. Advantages of a modified toluidine blue O stain and bronchoalveolar lavage for the diagnosis of Pneumocystis carinii pneumonia. *J Clin Microbiol.* 1985;22:803-807.

4. Grocott RGA. A stain for fungi. *Am J Clin Pathol.* 1955;25:975-979.

5. Chandler FW. Infectious disease pathology: morphologic and molecular approaches to diagnosis. *J Histotechnol.* 1995;18:183-186.

6. Grizzle WE. Theory and practice of silver staining in histopathology. *J Histotechnol.* 1996;19:183-195.

7. Churukian CJ, Schenk EA, Clark G. Pneumocystis carinii and fungi with ammoniacal silver. *Lab Med.* 1986;17:44-46.

8. Tome Y, Hayashi I, Matsuoka S, et al. A simple and highly reproducible staining method for fungi and other polysaccharide-rich microorganisms in animal tissues. *Stain Technol.* 1988;63:53-57.

9. Chandler FW, Watts IC. *Pathologic Diagnosis of Fungal Infections.* Chicago, IL: American Society of Clinical Pathologists; 1987: 56-57.

10. Huppert M, Oliver DJ, Sun SH. Combined methenamine-silver nitrate and hematoxylin & eosin stain for fungi in tissues. *J Clin Microbiol.* 1978;8:598-603.

11. Della Speranza V, Fail R. A common mistake when staining for fungi. *HistoLogic.* 2005;38:1-3.

12. Carson FL, Fredenburgh J, Maxwell JE. Inconsistent detection of Histoplasma capsulatum with periodic acid oxidation in the Grocott methenamine-silver nitrate (GMS) fungus stain. *J Histotechnol.* 1999;22:119-122.

13. Carson FL. *Histotechnology: A Self-Instructional Text.* 2nd ed. Chicago, IL: American Society of Clinical Pathologists; 1997: 196-197.

Trichrome Stains

Vinnie Della Speranza

The term *trichrome stain* refers to a group of related techniques utilized to distinguish various connective tissue elements, including collagen, striated and smooth muscle, erythrocytes, and fibrin. These methods employ three dyes, one of which may be a nuclear stain. Whereas immunohistochemical stains allow for identification of specific cell types, trichrome stains remain a useful screening tool for assessing changes in microscopic architecture associated with tissue pathology.

Trichrome stains are especially useful for assessing the presence and density of fibrosis in sections of liver, kidney, and lung. Identification of early fibrosis may allow for therapeutic intervention before end-stage disease. Early fibrosis may be inconspicuous or masked by an inflammatory infiltrate in the hematoxylin and eosin (H&E) stain; however, a well-differentiated trichrome stain is sufficiently sensitive to visualize early changes. Dense fibrosis, as confirmed by trichrome stain, is irreversible and reflects end-stage disease. Tumor invasion invokes a host reaction manifested by a mixture of fibrosis and inflammation known as *desmoplastic reaction*. Trichrome stains can highlight this reaction, especially in tissues where the surrounding stroma may be morphologically indistinguishable from desmoplasia in a routine H&E stain (eg, in uterine cervix and ovary).

Differential staining with trichrome methods is achieved by using two anionic dyes of contrasting color and widely different molecular sizes. This approach capitalizes on the observation that collagen always stains with the larger dye molecule, while muscle and cytoplasm stain with the smaller dye molecule. A number of popular trichrome stains can be found in classical histology texts; however, one can easily "invent" a trichrome stain by following the requirements of contrasting color and disparate molecular size[1] (Figures 10.1 and 10.2).

Among the various trichrome methods in use today, the following factors probably play a role in the staining process: (1) the physical properties of collagen and cytoplasm, (2) the manner in which large and small dye ions attach to tissue substrates, and (3) differences in amino acid composition of different tissue structures.[2] Tissue structures are believed to have different permeability after fixation, which seems most consistent with observed trichrome staining. In this model, formalin fix-

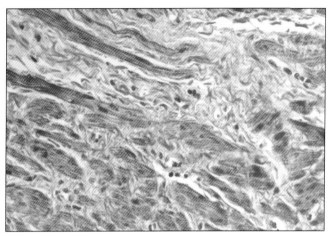

Figure 10.1. In this section stained with the Masson trichrome procedure, the red dye (small dye molecule) stains smooth muscle and rare erythrocytes, while aniline blue (large dye molecule) stains collagen.

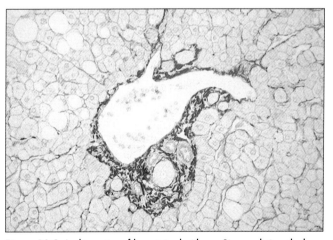

Figure 10.2. In this section of liver stained with van Gieson solution, the large dye molecule is red and stains the collagen previously stained blue in the Masson trichrome technique. The small dye molecule (picric acid) is yellow and stains both the smooth muscle and hepatocyte cytoplasm.

ation creates an insoluble protein network with greater porosity in collagen (especially Type IV) and much less so in muscle, erythrocytes, and cytoplasm.[3]

In practice, trichrome stains use two or more anionic dyes (those negatively charged in solution), applied individually (Masson, Mallory) or in combination (van

Gieson, Gomori), along with phosphotungstic acid (PTA) or phosphomolybdic acid (PMA), which some authors describe as behaving as an intermediate-sized "colorless dye."[2] When used in sequence, the smallest dye molecules will bind to cationic sites in all tissues but are easily washed from those that are more porous, making way for the largest dye molecules able to penetrate each structure. PTA or PMA are believed to displace small dye molecules from more porous tissues and are themselves replaced by the larger dye molecules.

Factors that affect trichrome staining results include fixative, pH, dye concentration (especially in combination dye solutions), and duration of tissue exposure to each solution. Neutral buffered formalin (10%) is routinely used by many laboratories as a general fixative to provide superior morphological preservation; however, by itself, formalin is inadequate to achieve good trichrome staining. Cross-linking fixatives, such as formaldehyde and gluteraldehyde, mask reactive chemical groups that would otherwise bind the acid dyes used in trichrome techniques. This phenomenon is especially true for tissues fixed in formalin for prolonged periods. Combination aldehyde fixatives containing metals are a better choice if formaldehyde must be used. Zinc formalin has been shown to provide satisfactory results.[4] Mercury-containing fixatives (such as B5 and Zenker) and Bouin solution, which contains picric acid, provide brilliant, intense trichrome staining.

Tissues fixed in formalin must be postfixed before undergoing trichrome staining. Postfixation is most often carried out with Bouin solution for 1 hour at room temperature or 15 minutes at 60°C. Mercury-containing solutions may also be used for postfixation, but it is important to note that this necessitates the subsequent removal of mercury pigment that would detract from the appearance of the stain. This removal is accomplished by exposing slides to an iodine solution, followed by sodium thiosulfate before the trichrome stain. Likewise, sections postfixed in Bouin solution should be thoroughly washed in tap water to remove all traces of picric acid before staining.

The pH plays an essential role in trichrome staining; the pH of the dye solution must be lowered, using acetic acid, to a level that is below the isoelectric point of tissue proteins. This pH level ensures that appropriate cationic (positively charged) binding sites will be accessible to the anionic dyes used in the trichrome stain. Trichrome staining is typically carried out at pH 2.5 or lower. Optimal trichrome staining with combination dye solutions occurs at pH 1.3; this low pH may be achieved with the addition of hydrochloric acid to the anionic dye solution.[3]

Dye concentration is especially important in techniques that use two or more dyes applied in a single solution, such as in the Gomori technique. A balance is essential to prevent one dye from overpowering the others, which can lead to inappropriate or nonspecific staining.

It should be noted that some nuclear stains, especially alum hematoxylins, will be easily removed by the acid pH of trichrome dye solutions; therefore, care must be taken to perform nuclear staining with dyes that are resistant to acidic environments, such as iron-mordanted hematoxylin. Several iron hematoxylin formulations, including Weigert, Lillie, and Verhoeff, are readily available to most laboratories and provide satisfactory results. Optimal nuclear staining is achieved when the working iron hematoxylin solution is prepared just before use. Crisp nuclear staining requires a thorough wash to remove excess hematoxylin dye. This process can be aided by a quick rinse in 70% ethanol before washing in tap water.[1]

Controls

As with most stains, the use of appropriate control tissue is of great benefit when performing trichrome stains. Smooth muscle in the wall of blood vessels is useful for verifying proper red staining; collagen, present in most tissues, is used to verify proper blue staining.

Unfortunately, it is quite easy to achieve suboptimal staining with trichrome methods, and a casual glance into the microscope revealing the presence of three colors can mislead one into believing appropriate staining has been achieved. Careful observation to identify appropriate coloration of the different tissue elements is essential to confirm successful staining.

What Should Be Seen in a Good Trichrome Stain

Masson Trichrome (Figures 10.3 and 10.4). The Masson trichrome method is perhaps the most commonly employed. In this technique, each of two anionic dyes is applied separately, with PMA or PTA as the intermediate step.

Nuclei	Blue-black
Cytoplasm, muscle, erythrocytes	Various shades of red
Collagen	Blue or green (depending on the collagen dye used)

Mallory Trichrome (Figure 10.5). This method uses three anionic dyes, the second and third combined with PTA and applied as one solution. This technique provides a wider differentiation of tissue structures and a more colorful result.[3]

Nuclei	Blue-black
Cytoplasm	Various shades of red, pink, and orange
Erythrocytes	Yellow to orange
Collagen	Blue

Gomori Trichrome (Figure 10.6). This method combines two anionic dyes (Chromotrope 2R and Fast Green FCF)

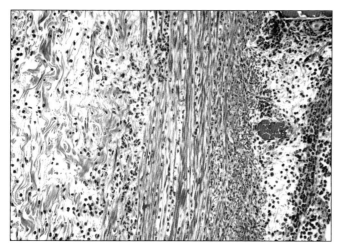

Figure 10.3. This section, stained with the Masson trichrome procedure using a blue counterstain, illustrates excellent staining intensity and contrast of various tissue elements. Nuclei are blue-black, muscle is red, collagen is blue, and red blood cells are bright red.

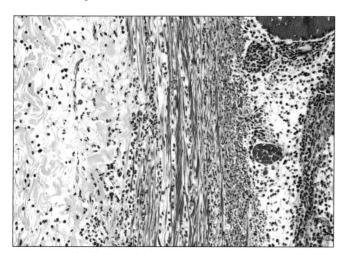

Figure 10.4. This duplicate of the section seen in Figure 10.3, stained with the Masson trichrome procedure using a green counterstain, illustrates excellent staining intensity and contrast of various tissue elements. Nuclei are blue-black, muscle is red, collagen is green, and red blood cells are bright red.

with PTA applied as one solution. When all of the dyes are applied at once, competition for the tissue-binding sites results in variations in color balance and stain intensity.[3]

Nuclei	Black
Cytoplasm, muscle	Red
Collagen	Blue or green

Van Gieson (Figure 10.7). A van Gieson counterstain, using acid fuchsin (red) and picric acid (yellow) combined in solution, can follow nuclear staining with iron hematoxylin.

Nuclei	Blue-black
Cytoplasm, muscle, erythrocytes	Yellow
Collagen	Red

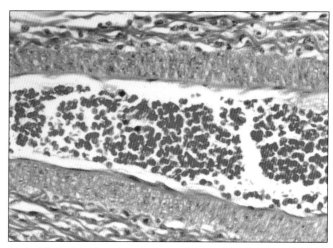

Figure 10.5. This section containing a muscular artery has been stained with the Mallory trichrome procedure and exhibits excellent differentiation of collagen, smooth muscle, and erythrocytes.

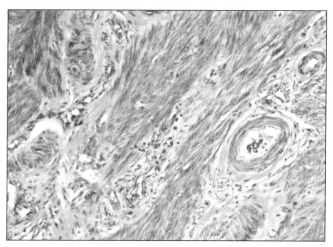

Figure 10.6. This section stained with the Gomori one-step trichrome procedure illustrates excellent differentiation among the various tissue elements.

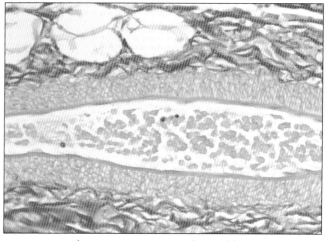

Figure 10.7. In the van Gieson staining procedure, acid fuchsin, the larger dye molecule, stains collagen fibers red; picric acid, the smaller dye molecule, stains erythrocytes, smooth muscle, and cytoplasm yellow.

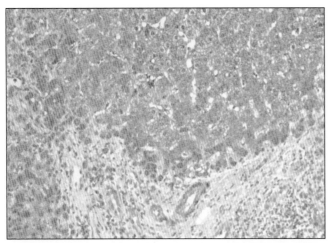

Figure 10.8. The nuclei in this section of liver stained with the Masson trichrome procedure are stained with the red dye, providing very poor contrast. Probably an alum hematoxylin was used. An acid-resistant nuclear stain, such as iron-mordant-ed hematoxylin, is required to withstand the acid pH of the dye solutions in this technique. Collagen staining is also inadequate in this section.

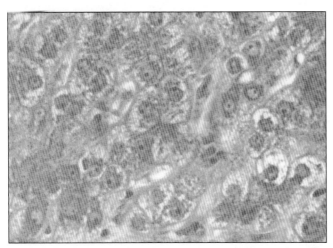

Figure 10.9. A high-magnification image of the section shown in Figure 10.8 stained with the Masson trichrome procedure illustrates the red staining of the hepatocyte nuclei.

Problems Encountered With Trichrome Stains

Many problems can be encountered with trichrome staining. Because the Gomori and Masson techniques are the most frequently used procedures, the problem-solving section will be devoted to those stains.

PROBLEM: Pale Nuclear Staining

APPEARANCE: Nuclei are pale and contrast poorly with the cytoplasm (Figures 10.8 and 10.9).

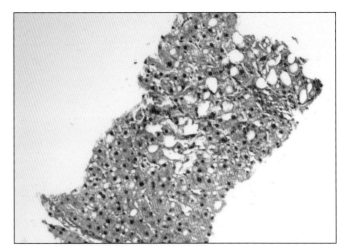

Figure 10.10. A needle core biopsy of liver stained with the Masson trichrome procedure exhibits overstained nuclei. Notice the grayish-blue coloration of cell cytoplasm, which should be red with this technique. When iron hematoxylin is improperly differentiated and incompletely washed from the section, red staining of cell cytoplasm will be compromised.

CAUSES:

• Iron-mordanted hematoxylin was not used for nuclear staining, and subsequent acidic dyes removed nuclear stain.

• Iron hematoxylin was not made fresh before use and became overoxidized; therefore, nuclear staining was incomplete.

• Insufficient time in nuclear stain led to weak staining.

• Counterstains are poorly differentiated, masking nuclear staining.

SOLUTIONS:

• Avoid the use of alum hematoxylins.

• Mix equal parts of iron hematoxylin stock solutions just before use to achieve intense nuclear staining.

• Determine optimal staining time in iron hematoxylin.

• Ensure proper differentiation of red and blue counter-stains.

PROBLEM: Poor Nuclear Detail; Nuclei Too Dark

APPEARANCE: Nuclei appear muddy and chromatin is dark and indistinct (Figures 10.10 and 10.11).

CAUSES:

• Section was overstained in iron hematoxylin.

• Insufficient washing occurred after nuclear staining in iron hematoxylin.

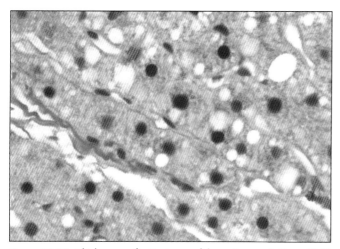

Figure 10.11. A higher-magnification image of the section seen in Figure 10.10 illustrates the overstained nuclei, which are very "smudgy" and exhibit no discernible chromatin pattern.

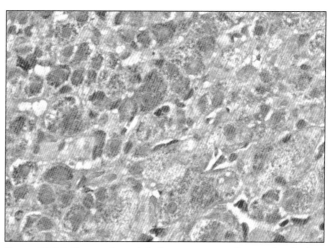

Figure 10.12. The cytoplasm of the hepatocytes is poorly stained in this liver section stained with the Masson trichrome procedure. The collagen is also not well stained, indicating that this section probably was not pretreated with picric acid before staining. Also, only rare nuclear staining can be seen.

SOLUTIONS:

- Determine optimal staining time in iron hematoxylin.

- Rinse quickly in 70% ethanol after the iron hematoxylin and follow with thorough washing in tap water.[1]

PROBLEM: Pale Staining With Cytoplasmic Dyes

APPEARANCE: There is lackluster staining, and tissue structures are faintly stained with red dye (Figures 10.12 and 10.13).

CAUSES:

- Prolonged water washes can remove cytoplasmic dyes.

- Prolonged exposure to alcohols during dehydration can remove cytoplasmic dyes.[5]

- Tissues fixed in formaldehyde without pretreatment before staining can cause this artifact.

- Use of old or overused reagents can cause this artifact.

- Tissue is autolyzed or fixation was delayed, resulting in poor preservation of tissues structures.

SOLUTIONS:

- Reduce wash times.

- Avoid prolonged times in dehydration solutions before mounting.

- Pretreat tissues fixed in formaldehyde with Bouin solution, picric acid solution, or mercuric chloride

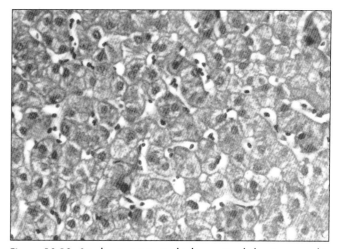

Figure 10.13. Cytoplasmic staining in this liver section lacks crispness and is somewhat overpowered by the collagen stain. This appearance is probably caused by overdifferentiation of the cytoplasmic dye.

solution to achieve desired mordanting before staining.

- Use the cytoplasmic dye solutions no more than twice.

COMMENTS: Inadequately preserved tissues will typically yield suboptimal trichrome staining. The detrimental effects of autolyzed or poorly preserved tissue cannot be corrected.

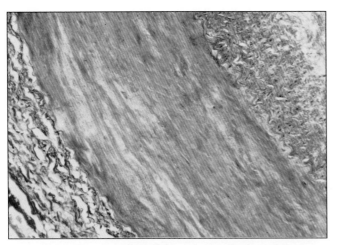

Figure 10.14. This section of a muscular artery stained with a trichrome procedure demonstrates minimal red staining of the smooth muscle. The red dye is probably old or overused and should be replaced.

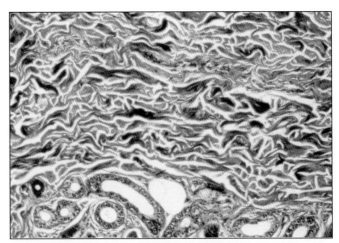

Figure 10.16. A section of skin illustrating the artifact of uptake of the red dye by collagen. Pathologically altered collagen may cause this type of staining, as will inadequate differentiation of the red dye or poor microtomy techniques.

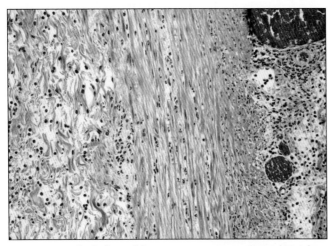

Figure 10.15. This duplicate of the sections seen in Figures 10.3 and 10.4 shows pinkish-grey staining of the smooth muscle, even though erythrocytes are brilliantly stained. This section was not pretreated before staining with the Masson trichrome procedure.

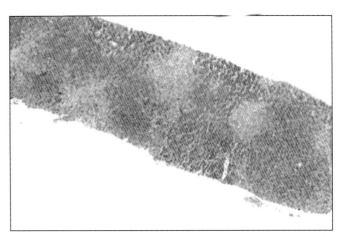

Figure 10.17. In this low-magnification image of a needle biopsy of liver, the staining of nuclei and collagen is notably absent, and the stain appears very uneven.

SOLUTIONS:

- Adjust time in iron hematoxylin.
- Wash thoroughly after iron hematoxylin using 70% ethanol and water.
- Change reagents.
- Pretreat tissues fixed in formaldehyde with Bouin solution, picric acid solution, or mercuric chloride solution to achieve desired mordanting before staining.

COMMENTS: Overstaining with iron hematoxylin will cause this dye to adhere to structures other than nuclei.

PROBLEM: Muscle Unstained or Grey Rather Than Red

APPEARANCE: The muscle is unstained or grey and has not taken up the red dye (Figures 10.14 and 10.15).

CAUSES:

- Overstaining occurred with iron hematoxylin, or there was inadequate removal of unbound iron hematoxylin.
- Old or depleted reagents were used.
- Tissues were fixed in formaldehyde without pretreatment before staining.

PROBLEM: Uneven or Incorrect Staining

APPEARANCE: Tissue structures exhibit the wrong color or uneven staining (Figures 10.16 and 10.17).

CAUSES:

- Tissues were fixed in formaldehyde without postfixation before staining.
- Tissues were improperly differentiated.
- The pH of one or more of the staining solutions is incorrect.
- There was improper washing in acetic acid solution.
- Tissues were frozen and thawed before fixation.
- Trichrome staining was carried out in a microwave device.

SOLUTIONS:

- Postfix tissues fixed in formaldehyde with Bouin solution, picric acid solution, or mercuric chloride solution to achieve desired mordanting before staining.
- Proper differentiation requires accurate timing of each step in the staining procedure. Avoid prolonged washes in acetic acid solution, which will remove dyes from desired structures.
- Verify that the pH of the dye solutions is 2.5 or lower.
- Avoid using tissues that were frozen before trichrome staining. Freezing and thawing of tissues before fixation appears to alter their porosity to various dyes, which may allow larger dyes to penetrate structures that they typically would not.[2]
- Reduce the staining temperature. Structures staining an unexpected color can result when procedures are accelerated in a microwave device. Reduce the temperature or staining time of the second acid dye step,[5] but keep in mind that pathologically altered collagen may also bind the red dyes.[6]

COMMENTS: When unexpected colors are obtained, consider the following possibilities:

- If sections display a yellowish tinge, verify that sections were adequately washed after pretreatment with Bouin or picric acid solutions.
- Color balance may be altered by pH or staining times, especially in one-step trichrome methods. If staining is too red, verify that the pH of the staining solution is 2.0 or less. If necessary, adjust the pH downward with 0.1 M hydrochloric acid[5]; if the pH is correct, consider altering staining times.

References

1. Della Speranza V. Trichrome staining: concepts and pitfalls. In: *HQIP: A Final Critique.* Northfield, IL: College of American Pathologists; 2003: 23-27.

2. Kiernan JA. *Histological and Histochemical Methods: Theory and Practice.* 3rd ed. Oxford, England: Butterworth Heinemann; 1999: 150-156.

3. Tunnicliffe J. Trichrome techniques. In: *HQIP: A Final Critique.* Northfield, IL: College of American Pathologists; 2006: 1-5-education.

4. Churukian CJ. *Manual of the Special Stains Laboratory.* Rochester, NY: University of Rochester Medical Center; 1997.

5. Horobin R, Bancroft J. *Troubleshooting Histology Stains.* New York, NY: Churchill Livingstone; 2000: 68-70, 114-117.

6. Vacca LL. *Laboratory Manual of Histochemistry.* New York, NY: Raven Press; 1985: 308-310.

Reticulin

Lena T. Spencer

Reticular fibers are small in diameter, resist dyes, and are difficult to demonstrate with routine hematoxylin and eosin (H&E) staining. They can be demonstrated by some dyes that will color the fibers, although most of these staining methods do not visualize the fine fibers very well. Because reticular fibers are argyrophilic ("silver loving"), the metallic impregnation techniques will demonstrate reticular fibers in a more striking manner and are universally accepted as the method of choice.

Reticular fiber "staining" is dependent upon the reactive groups present in the carbohydrate matrix in which the fibers are embedded and not upon the fibrillar elements. The principle of the silver reaction is very similar to that of the periodic acid–Schiff reaction; the adjacent glycol groups of the hexose sugars in the carbohydrate matrix of the reticulin are oxidized to aldehydes.[1] Reticular fibers have a low natural affinity for silver salts, requiring suitable pretreatment to enhance the selectivity of the impregnation.[2] Ammoniacal silver reactions require oxidation (eg, with potassium permanganate or periodic acid), which enhances subsequent staining, and sensitization with a metallic salt (eg, uranyl nitrate, ferric ammonium sulfate, or dilute silver nitrate), which begins the impregnation of reticular fibers. These steps are followed by the application of the ammoniacal silver complex (diamine silver), which replaces the sensitizing metal that has impregnated the reticulin fibers. The ammoniacal silver solution employs concentrated ammonium hydroxide (a strong base), which is added to an aqueous solution of silver nitrate at pH 5.0; addition of the base immediately raises the pH of the silver nitrate solution to 9.5, producing a brown-black precipitate of silver hydroxide. Additional ammonium hydroxide is then added to the solution to produce gradual clearing of the precipitate by the formation of a silver diamine complex. Finally, a small amount of ammonium hydroxide is added to raise the pH to 11 to 12. At this point, the concentration of the silver diamine complex is high, the concentration of silver ions is low, and the solution is ready to use.[1] Because the diamine silver solution has a very high pH (11 to 12), it may cause tissue detachment. Further deposition of silver occurs when incompletely washed sections are placed in a reducing solution (formaldehyde). Metallic silver is then converted to metallic gold by the use of a toning reagent (gold chloride), providing stability, contrast, and clarity. Unreduced silver and gold are removed by sodium thiosulfate in order to prevent subsequent nonspecific reduction of silver by exposure to light. The tissue may be counterstained with nuclear fast red, light green, or fast green, if desired.[3] Although there are many modifications, most rely on the same chemical principles and vary primarily in the choice of oxidizer, sensitizer, and preparation of the diamine silver solution.

Application

The pattern of reticular fibers can be helpful in the diagnosis of certain types of tumors. For example, in most carcinomas, reticulin surrounds nests of tumor cells, whereas in sarcomas, the reticulin pattern is more mesh-like, surrounding individual cells. Other diseases with a characteristic reticular pattern include hepatocellular fibrosis, cirrhosis, and necrotic liver disease. In renal biopsies, reticulin stains may show abnormalities of glomerular basement membranes. In chronic myeloproliferative diseases, such as chronic myelogenous leukemia, an increase in the amount of reticulin in the bone marrow generally correlates with an increased number of megakaryocytes, larger spleen size, and more severe anemia as hematopoietic elements are replaced by reticular fibrosis.

Controls

The best control for reticulin staining is a well-processed section of liver.

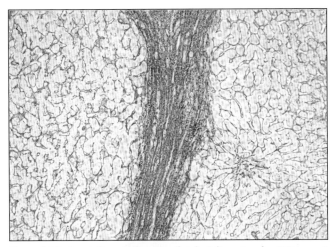

Figure 11.1. A reticulin-stained section of cirrhotic liver viewed at 100x magnification. The reticulin fibers are well demonstrated and easily discerned at this magnification. Nuclear fast red has been used as the counterstain.

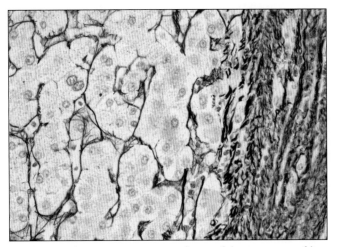

Figure 11.2. This image is a 450x magnification of the same section of liver seen in Figure 11.1. Note the specificity of the stain and the total lack of nonspecific staining.

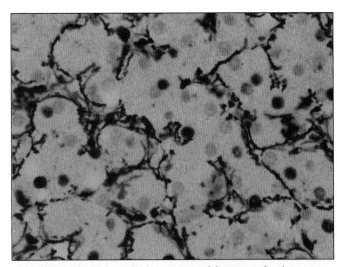

Figure 11.3. The nuclei in this liver section exhibit nonspecific silver staining, which may be the result of using improperly cleaned glassware.

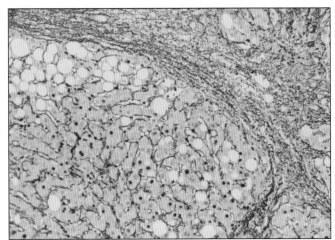

Figure 11.4. Silver is deposited throughout this section of liver, obscuring delicate details. This appearance could be the result of using metal instruments to transfer slides during the staining process.

What Should Be Seen in a Good Reticulin Stain

Well-stained reticulin exhibits well-defined, linear black fibers. No background, beading effect, or nuclear staining should be seen. The nuclei and other tissue elements should stain the color of the chosen counterstain. To determine whether the reticulin is well demonstrated, the slide should be microscopically examined with the 10x objective; a well-defined pattern should be seen at this magnification (Figure 11.1). A higher magnification may be used to view the finer reticulin fibers (Figure 11.2).

Problems Encountered With the Reticulin Stain

PROBLEM: Nonspecific Silver Staining

APPEARANCE: There is an unexpected grayish appearance to all tissue elements or a tiny black granular precipitate on or around the tissue section (Figures 11.3, 11.4, and 11.5).

CAUSES:

- Improperly cleaned glassware was used.
- Metal instruments were used during the preparation of the silver reagents.

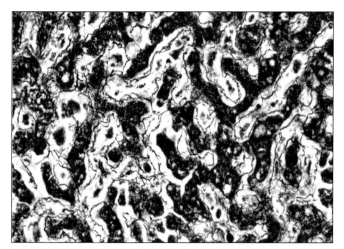

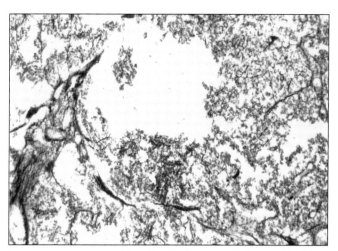

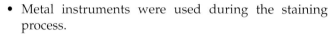

Figure 11.5. Marked nonspecific staining of the liver parenchyma is seen in this reticulin-stained slide. The pH of the impregnating solution was below 11.

Figure 11.6. A section of lymph node showing marked tissue detachment caused by the high pH of the diamine silver solution. Hematoxylin was used as the counterstain.

- Metal instruments were used during the staining process.
- The tissue was fixed in a heavy-metal–containing fixative.
- The pH of the impregnating solution was below 11.0.

SOLUTIONS:

- Use chemically cleaned glassware; chemical cleaners include concentrated nitric acid, bleach, and commercial glass cleaner.
- Use freshly prepared reagents.
- Use plastic or coated instruments when staining and preparing solutions.
- Use a different fixative, one that does not include a heavy metal.
- Use high-quality water in all steps of the procedure, including the preparation of solutions.

PROBLEM: Tissue Sections Detaching From the Slide

APPEARANCE: The tissue section is partially or completely missing from the slide (Figures 11.6 and 11.7).

CAUSES:

- The pH of the silver solution is too high.
- The silver solution was overheated.

SOLUTIONS:

- Use positively charged or coated slides (some adhesive additives may cause background staining on the slide).

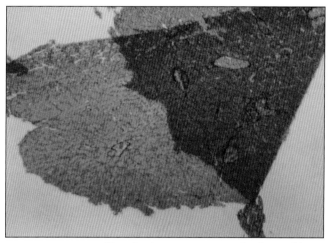

Figure 11.7. A section of liver that demonstrates extreme detachment of the tissue. The fold may obscure important diagnostic areas of the slide. Noncharged slides were used.

- Properly drain and dry slides before staining.
- Carefully monitor the temperature of the silver solution.

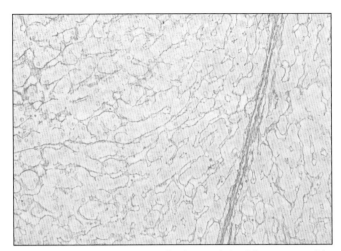

Figure 11.8. The reticulin fibers are faintly stained; the slide is not optimal for diagnosis. Slides were removed from solution before the optimal end point was achieved.

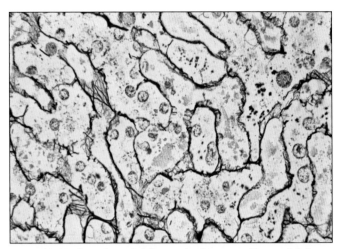

Figure 11.10. The nuclei are lightly stained in this section of liver, and slight precipitate can also be seen. No counterstain was used. Microscopic evaluation during each step in the process can prevent such problems.

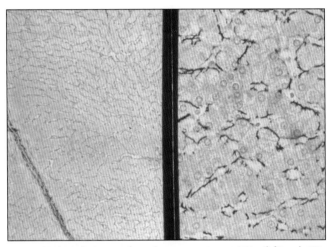

Figure 11.9. A dual image from the same section, at 100x (left) and 450x (right) magnifications. The reticulin is only partially stained, showing a broken pattern. This appearance may be the result of using old or outdated ammonium hydroxide to prepare the silver solution.

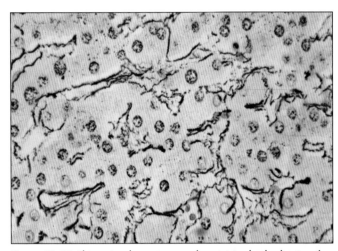

Figure 11.11. This section demonstrates nuclear staining by the diamine silver solution, but no other nonspecific staining can be seen. Nuclear fast red was used as the counterstain.

PROBLEM: Incomplete Impregnation of Reticulin Fibers

APPEARANCE: Reticulin fibers stain gray rather than a crisp black; the fibers may appear broken or discontinuous when viewed microscopically (Figures 11.8 and 11.9).

CAUSES:

- Old or weak ammonium hydroxide was used in the preparation of the silver solution.
- Reagents were not freshly prepared.
- Slides were removed from the impregnating solution too soon.

SOLUTIONS:

- Use a new bottle of ammonium hydroxide to prepare the silver solution.
- Microscopically evaluate the end point of the reaction.

COMMENTS: Check to see that the final ammoniacal silver solution has visible granules or slight turbidity. The ammonium hydroxide may be old or weak as a result of the gas coming out of solution, which should be apparent because more than the usual amount of ammonium hydroxide will be required to prepare the ammoniacal silver solution. Excess ammonium hydroxide added to the solution impairs impregnation of the reticular fibers, which may result in weak staining.

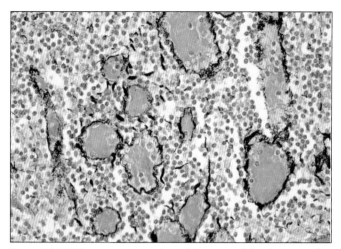

Figure 11.12. This section shows a beaded deposition of the silver, an artifact that occurs when old uranyl nitrate solution is used in the reticulin stain.

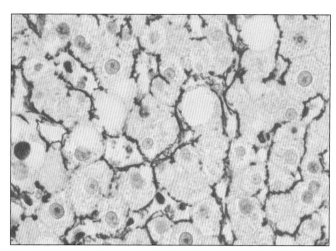

Figure 11.13. The silver patterning lacks the fine continuous line of well-stained reticulin fibers. The tissue is slightly overstained, with silver deposits making the fibers look discontinuous.

PROBLEM: Nuclei Excessively Stained With Silver

APPEARANCE: The pattern of silver deposition varies from black granules in the nuclei to solid black nuclei (Figures 11.10 and 11.11).

CAUSES:

- There was prolonged exposure to the sensitizing metallic salt solution.[4]
- The temperature was too high during impregnation.

SOLUTIONS:

- Reduce the time in the sensitizer.[4]
- Acidify the oxidizer when using potassium permanganate; use 2.5 mL of 3% sulfuric acid to 47.5 mL of 0.5% potassium permanganate.
- Carefully monitor the temperature of the silver solution.

PROBLEM: Granular, Rather Than Linear, Deposition of Silver on the Reticulin Fibers

APPEARANCE: The reticular fibers look like strings of pearls, rather than fine continuous lines (Figures 11.12 and 11.13).

CAUSES:

- Old uranyl nitrate was used.
- Old ammonium hydroxide was used.

SOLUTIONS:

- Prepare a new solution of uranyl nitrate.
- Use a new bottle of ammonium hydroxide when preparing solutions.

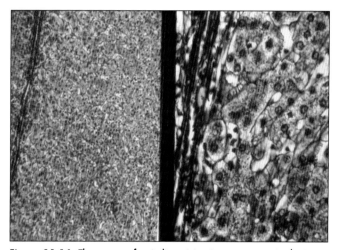

Figure 11.14. The pattern of reticulin staining is not apparent in the image taken at 100x magnification (left); however, at 450x magnification (right) the reticulin fibers can be seen. Although the reticulin is well stained, the counterstain is masking some of the finer fibers.

PROBLEM: Section Is Over-Counterstained or Poor Choice of Counterstain

APPEARANCE: The counterstain is dark enough to mask the silver-stained reticulin fibers, or there is a decrease in contrast between tissue structures (Figure 11.14).

CAUSE:

- The tissue section remained too long in the counterstain.

SOLUTIONS:

- Decrease the time in the counterstain.
- Do not use a counterstain.

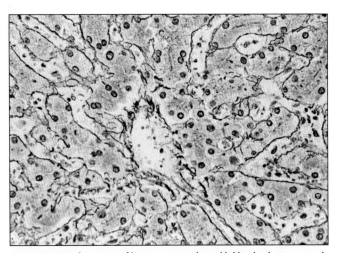

Figure 11.15. This section of liver is overtoned in gold chloride; the tissue is pale violet-gray. Reticulin fibers are not crisp and are difficult to distinguish from the surrounding tissue elements. The light green counterstain is adequate for the stain.

PROBLEM: Section Overtoned in Gold Chloride

APPEARANCE: The tissue has a grey, nonspecific coloration, with very light staining (Figure 11.15).

CAUSE:

• Slides were not removed from the gold chloride at the appropriate time.

SOLUTIONS:

• Check slides microscopically during the staining process.

• Carefully control the time slides are exposed to the gold chloride solution.

References

1. Sheehan DC, Hrapchak BB. *Theory and Practice of Histotechnology.* St Louis, MO: CV Mosby; 1980: 180-188.

2. Bancroft JD, Gamble M. *Theory and Practice of Histological Techniques.* 5th ed. New York, NY: Churchill Livingstone; 1996: 158-159.

3. Carson, FL. *Histotechnology: A Self-Instructional Text.* 2nd ed. Chicago, IL: American Society of Clinical Pathologists; 1997: 143-147.

4. Horobin RW, Bancroft, JD. *Troubleshooting Histology Stains.* New York, NY: Churchill Livingstone; 1998: 72-75.

Elastin Stains

Freida L. Carson

Elastin, one of the connective tissue fibers, is an extracellular, insoluble polymeric protein with a rubber-like consistency (molecular weight of 70 kilodaltons) that gives elasticity to tissues and organs. It is found abundantly in those tissues requiring great flexibility, thus allowing recovery of tissue shape after normal deformation or stretching. It is especially prominent in the walls of arteries and in the lungs, intestines, urinary bladder, and skin. Because elastic tissue is relatively stable, the body stops making elastin once it reaches maturity soon after puberty. There are three stages of elastic fiber development. The first stage is formation of oxytalan fibers, which are initially resistant to tension but become progressively elastic with continued development to maturity. These fibers will not stain with aldehyde fuchsin unless previously oxidized with potassium permanganate, performic acid, or peracetic acid. They have also been reported to remain unstained with the Verhoeff-van Gieson technique, with or without prior oxidation.[1,2] The second stage involves the formation of elaunin fibers by an irregular deposition of the protein elastin between the oxytalan fibers. Elaunin fibers are found in the dermis and around sweat glands and will stain with orcein, aldehyde fuchsin, and resorcin-fuchsin without prior oxidation; they will not stain with the Verhoeff technique.[1] In the third stage, elastin gradually accumulates, until it occupies the center of each fiber bundle, which then is surrounded by a thin sheath of microfibrils to become true elastic fibers.[1] Elastic fibers can vary in diameter from about 1 to 4 µm and can only be seen on hematoxylin-and-eosin (H&E)–stained sections when arranged in thick sheets.

Elastic stains are useful in the identification of tumor invasion of large blood vessels and pleura, for evaluating arteriovenous malformations and aneurysms, and for demonstrating disruption of the elastic tissue in cases of emphysema. There have been several reports that routine elastic stains are very useful and practical in evaluating the venous invasion status in colorectal cancer, and implementation in routine pathology practice was recommended to improve patient care.[3,4] Some cases of vasculitis require elastic stains to either confirm that an artery is present or to look for evidence of previous dam-

age; and when paired with a nuclear counterstain, the elastic stain can clearly demonstrate vascular destruction. Renal pathologists sometimes use elastic stains for evaluating vasculitis as well.

Stains for elastic fibers can be separated into four groups, which are modifications of the following four methods: (1) Verhoeff hematoxylin, (2) orcein, (3) Weigert resorcin-fuchsin, and (4) aldehyde fuchsin. In addition, elastic fibers will stain selectively at high pH (up to pH 10) with eosin B and Biebrich scarlet and at low pH with Victoria blue 4R.[5] Elastic fibers are weakly birefringent and exhibit yellowish autofluorescence. For specific identification, elastase, a pancreatic enzyme, can be used to digest elastin.

The Verhoeff hematoxylin methods are the most widely used in clinical laboratory practice for the identification of elastic fibers because they are fast, and, when paired with the van Gieson counterstain (Verhoeff-van Gieson stain), they provide a good overall assessment of connective tissue elements. This classical method also works well after all of the routine fixatives. Verhoeff hematoxylin is a mixture of alcoholic hematoxylin, ferric chloride, and iodine, which produces a thick, black, almost syrupy staining solution. Iodine and ferric chloride serve as both mordants and oxidizing agents in the staining solution. It is the oxidizing property of these two reagents that probably accounts for the production of the black dye, which possesses cationic properties, as well as converting the hematoxylin to hematein. The iodine also may serve as a dye-trapping agent, retarding the loss of hematein from elastic fibers in the subsequent differentiation step.[6]

Because the stain has no defined end point, this differentiation step is critical for achieving reproducible results, and some experience and expertise are necessary. Finer fibers will not be demonstrated when the stain is overdifferentiated.

Perhaps the simplest group of staining methods for displaying elastic fibers is the orcein group. Along with simplicity, these methods share with the resorcin-fuchsin techniques a remarkable selectivity for elastic tissue. Orcein, originally a vegetable dye, has now been synthesized and is commercially available. The staining solu-

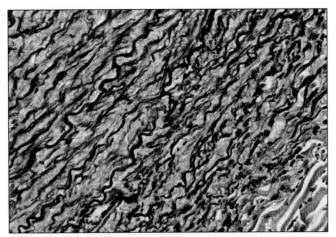

Figure 12.1. This section of aorta is stained with the Verhoeff-van Gieson technique. The elastic fibers are well differentiated, with some fine fibers visible. The collagen and smooth muscle are also differentially stained with the van Gieson counterstain.

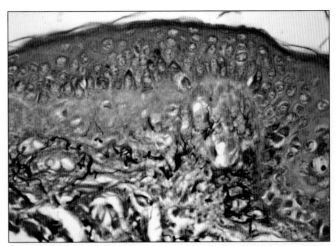

Figure 12.3. This section of skin is stained with the resorcin-fuchsin technique and counterstained with van Gieson solution. There is excellent contrast between the elastic fibers and the background, with similarity to the Verhoeff-van Gieson technique. (Image courtesy of Peggy Wenk, William Beaumont Hospital, Royal Oaks, Michigan.)

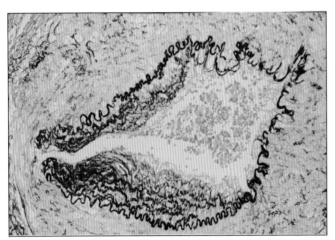

Figure 12.2. This small blood vessel is stained with the orcein technique. There is excellent contrast between the elastic fibers and the background.

tion of orcein consists of 1% synthetic orcein dissolved in warm 70% alcohol, to which is added 1.0 mL of concentrated hydrochloric acid. This simple solution shows a spectacular affinity for elastic tissue and stains it a deep brown. Although the precise mechanism of orcein binding to elastic fibers is not clear, van der Waals forces are thought to be involved.

Another important group of elastin stains are the iron resorcin lakes of basic fuchsin and other basic dyes. These methods tend to be slow and the solutions are time consuming and tedious to prepare, but when prepared correctly, they show remarkable selectivity for elastic fibers and demonstrate fine fibers very well.[7] The resorcin-fuchsin solution is actually a complex formed by combining a hot basic fuchsin and resorcin dye solution with ferric chloride, rendering an iron

resorcin lake of the basic fuchsin. It is this complex that attaches to the elastic fibers and stains them blue-black. Although the mechanism of the binding of the stain is not fully understood, it is generally thought that formation of hydrogen bonds between some part of the elastic tissue and the phenol groups of the resorcin-fuchsin complex is responsible for staining. Although differentiation is involved in this method, the likelihood of overdifferentiation is very small, as compared with the Verhoeff hematoxylin methods.

The final group consists of the aldehyde fuchsin methods, introduced by Gomori in 1950 for staining both coarse and fine elastic fibers.[8] These are less selective than the other methods, demonstrating other tissue components similarly, including beta cells of the pancreas, hepatitis B surface antigen, gastric chief cells, and granules of both mast cells and pituitary basophils. The staining solution is prepared by the addition of hydrochloric acid and "fresh" paraldehyde to basic fuchsin in an alcohol solution. Paraldehyde increases the depth of staining by linking with basic fuchsin and forming aldehyde fuchsin. The aldehyde and fuchsin together form Schiff bases, which have an unexplained affinity for elastic fibers and stain them deep purple. Various counterstains have been used with aldehyde fuchsin; however, fast green or light green contrast best with the deep purple primary dye.

Controls

Although sections of aorta are most frequently used as a control for elastic stains, it is better to use a smaller muscular artery because the demonstration of the fine elastic

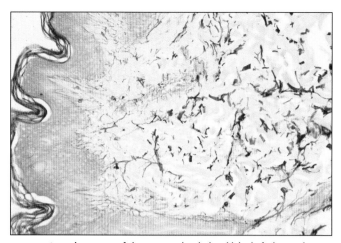

Figure 12.4. This section of skin is stained with the aldehyde fuchsin technique. A light green counterstain has been used and provides an excellent contrast to the purple elastic fibers.

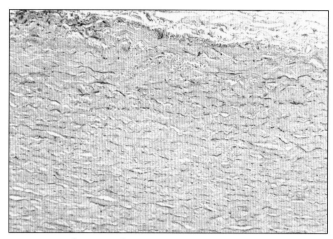

Figure 12.5. This section of aorta is stained with the Verhoeff-van Gieson technique. Elastic fibers have been markedly over-decolorized and only rare, black-stained fibers can be seen.

fibers within the muscular wall can better determine the end point of differentiation. It is very easy to overdifferentiate sections of aorta and not be aware of it.

What Should Be Seen in a Good Stain for Elastic Fibers

Regardless of the technique used, the elastic fibers (including fine fibers) should be well stained and contrast well with the counterstain used. The counterstain should enhance the fiber staining and should never reduce the contrast. No staining artifacts should be present. Good elastic stains by the various techniques are demonstrated in Figures 12.1 through 12.4.

Problems Encountered With the Verhoeff Technique

PROBLEM: Pale Staining of Elastic Fibers

APPEARANCE: The elastic fibers are very pale and do not contrast well with the background (Figures 12.5 and 12.6).

CAUSES:

- Verhoeff hematoxylin solution was incorrectly prepared.
- Verhoeff hematoxylin solution is too old.
- Section is over-decolorized.

SOLUTIONS:

- Ensure that the Verhoeff hematoxylin solution is correctly prepared. The reagents must be mixed in the proper order.
- Prepare fresh Verhoeff hematoxylin solution. This solution does not age well. Bradbury and Rae indicate that, although most texts state that the solution

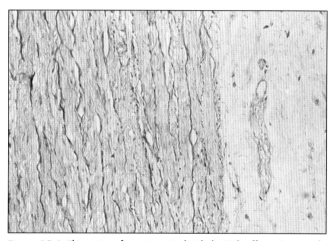

Figure 12.6. This section of aorta is stained with the Verhoeff-van Gieson technique. The elastic fibers have been moderately over-decolorized and only larger, black-stained fibers can be seen.

should be used within 2 to 3 hours, they have successfully used it up to 48 hours.[2]

- Decolorize each slide microscopically. Do not time the differentiation step by the control slide. Because further decolorization will occur in the van Gieson counterstain, the section should be left slightly under-decolorized in the ferric chloride solution.
- Restain the section. Overdifferentiated sections may be restained at any point provided they have not been in alcohol.

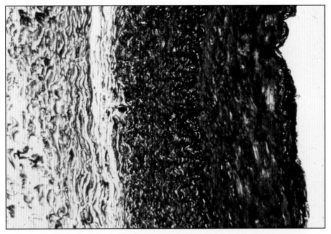

Figure 12.7. This section of aorta is stained with the Verhoeff-van Gieson technique. The elastic fibers have been markedly under-decolorized and are difficult to distinguish from the background.

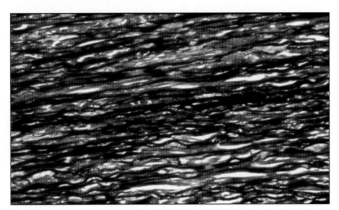

Figure 12.8. This section of aorta is stained with the Verhoeff–van Gieson technique. The elastic fibers have been markedly under-decolorized and are difficult to distinguish from the background and from each other.

PROBLEM: Background Stained With Verhoeff Hematoxylin

APPEARANCE: The background is stained blue-gray and the elastic fibers do not contrast with the background (Figures 12.7 and 12.8).

CAUSE:

- The section has been under-decolorized.

SOLUTIONS:

- Leave the section in the ferric chloride solution for a longer period of time.
- Check the differentiation step on each slide microscopically. Do not time the differentiation step by the control section.

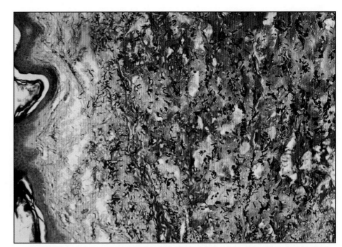

Figure 12.9. Although the contrast between the elastic fibers and the counterstain is satisfactory, the van Gieson counterstain in this Verhoeff-van Gieson stain is very poor. The picric acid used to make the van Gieson stain was not saturated, and therefore the correct staining of collagen is not seen; collagen should be stained red, as shown in Figure 12.1.

PROBLEM: Poor Counterstain or Deficient Contrast

APPEARANCE: The collagen and muscle are not differentially stained, or the elastic fibers do not contrast well with the background (Figures 12.9 and 12.10).

CAUSES:

- The picric acid used to prepare the van Gieson stain was not a saturated solution.
- Differentiation of the elastic fibers may be inadequate.

SOLUTIONS:

- Ensure that the picric acid solution used in the preparation of the van Gieson stain is saturated.
- Ensure that the elastic fibers are properly differentiated.

Problems Encountered With the Orcein Technique

PROBLEM: Poor Staining of Elastic Fibers

APPEARANCE: The elastic fibers are not well stained and do not contrast with the background (Figure 12.11).

CAUSE:

- The synthetic dye lot is bad.

SOLUTION:

- Use only dyes certified by the Biological Stain Commission for the preparation of the staining solution.

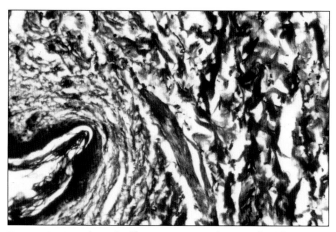

Figure 12.10. In this Verhoeff-van Gieson–stained section, the differentiation of the elastic fibers is incomplete, and there is iron hematoxylin stain in the background. The van Gieson stain is also very poor, and the correct differentiation between collagen and muscle is not seen; muscle should be yellow and collagen should be red.

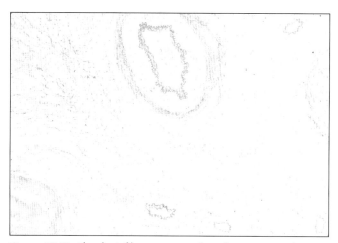

Figure 12.11. The elastic fibers are very pale in this orcein-stained section. Compare this staining with the excellent staining of the fibers seen in Figure 12.2.

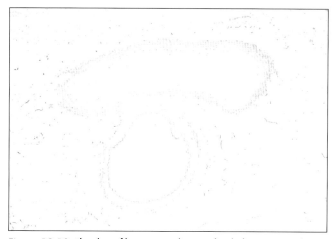

Figure 12.12. The elastic fibers are poorly stained with the resorcin technique in this tissue section.

Problems Encountered With the Weigert Resorcin-Fuchsin Technique

PROBLEM: Elastic Fibers Not Stained Well After an Extended Period in the Dye Solution

APPEARANCE: The elastic fibers are either pale or unstained (Figure 12.12).

CAUSES:

- The staining solution was prepared poorly.
- There are impurities in the ferric chloride. Some ferrous salt is present in fresh ferric chloride, so ferric nitrate is a better salt for use.[2]
- The composition of basic fuchsin is variable, with at least three dyes present in many batches. This variable composition will affect both the staining and storage properties of the solution.[2]

SOLUTIONS:

- Follow the instructions exactly for the preparation of the dye solution. A good solution can be used for several months.
- Use certified dyes.
- Substitute ferric nitrate for the ferric chloride if there are problems with the solution.

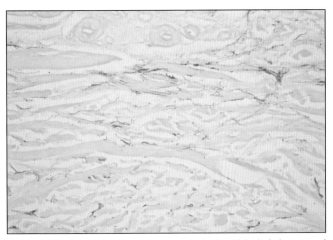

Figure 12.13. The elastic fibers are very pale in this aldehyde fuchsin-stained section and do not contrast with the light green–stained background.

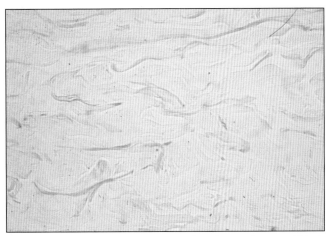

Figure 12.14. The elastic fibers are severely understained in this aldehyde fuchsin-stained section of skin, resulting in practically no contrast between the fibers and the background.

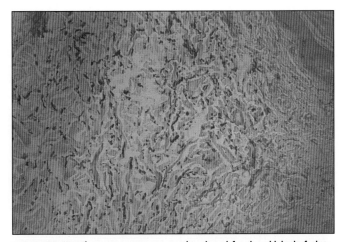

Figure 12.15. The counterstain was poorly selected for this aldehyde fuchsin-stained section of skin, and the contrast is extremely poor. A light green counterstain would provide a better contrast.

Problems Encountered With the Aldehyde Fuchsin Technique

PROBLEM: Inadequate Staining of Elastic Fibers

APPEARANCE: Elastic fibers are either very pale or unstained (Figures 12.13 and 12.14).

CAUSES:

- Solution has not been sufficiently ripened.
- Solution is too old.

SOLUTIONS:

- Ensure that the solution is sufficiently ripened.
- Prepare the solution with basic fuchsin that is mainly pararosaniline. Solutions prepared from basic fuchsin that is mainly rosaniline will not stain some substances that are reported to stain with aldehyde fuchsin.[9]
- Ensure that the paraldehyde used in the preparation of the staining solution is from a freshly opened vial. Acetaldehyde, a much cheaper reagent, may be substituted for paraldehyde, but four times the quantity must be used.[10]

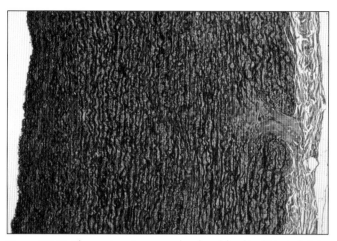

Figure 12.16. The counterstain was poorly selected for this aldehyde fuchsin-stained section of aorta, and the contrast is extremely poor. A light green counterstain would provide a better contrast.

PROBLEM: Poor Contrast

APPEARANCE: The elastic fibers do not contrast well with the background.

CAUSES:

- The elastic fibers are pale (refer again to Figures 12.13 and 12.14).

- There is a poor choice of counterstain (Figure 12.15 and 12.16).

SOLUTIONS:

- Ensure that the elastic fibers are correctly stained.

- Change counterstains. Light green provides the best contrast for the aldehyde fuchsin stain, although van Gieson, eosin, and nuclear fast red are also recommended.[2]

References

1. Ellis RC. Connective tissue. In: Woods, Ellis RC. *Laboratory Histopathology: A Complete Reference.* New York, NY: Churchill Livingstone; 1994.

2. Bradbury P, Rae K. Connective tissues and staining. In: Bancroft JD, Stevens A, eds. *Theory and Practice of Histological Techniques.* 4th ed. New York, NY: Churchill Livingstone; 1996: 117-134.

3. Vass DG, Ainsworth JH, Anderson DM, Foulis AK. The value of an elastic tissue stain in detecting venous invasion in colorectal cancer. *J Clin Pathol.* 2004;57:769-772.

4. Abdulkader M, Abdulla K, Rakha E, Kaye P. Routine elastic staining assists detection of vascular invasion in colorectal cancer. *Histopathology.* 2006;49:487-492.

5. Lyon H, Hoyer PE, Prento P. Proteins. In: Lyon H, ed. *Theory and Strategy in Histochemistry.* Berlin, Germany: Springer-Verlag; 1991.

6. Thompson SW. *Selected Histochemical and Histopathological Methods.* Springfield, IL: Charles C. Thomas; 1966.

7. Bancroft JD, Cook HC. *Manual of Histological Techniques and Their Diagnostic Application.* New York, NY: Churchill Livingstone; 1994: 54-62.

8. Gomori G. Aldehyde-fuchsin: a new stain for elastic tissue. *Am J Clin Pathol.* 1950;20:665-666.

9. Mowry RW. Aldehyde fuchsin staining, direct or after oxidation: problems and remedies, with special reference to human pancreatic B cells, pituitaries and elastic fibers. *Stain Technol.* 1978;53:141-154.

10. Carson FL. *Histotechnology: A Self-Instructional Text.* 2nd ed. Chicago, IL: American Society of Clinical Pathologists; 1997: 141.

Basement Membrane

Lena T. Spencer

The basement membrane (BM) is an amorphous, extracellular support layer forming an interface between the epithelium and underlying connective tissue. With special stains, the BM appears as a continuous layer closely associated with the base of the epithelium and varies in thickness, depending on the site. The BM is not a single structural entity but consists of three distinct components: the lamina rara (lucida), lamina densa, and lamina reticularis. The lamina lucida is adjacent to the surface cells and consists primarily of carbohydrate complexes. The lamina densa consists of a meshwork of fibrils, primarily Type IV collagen, surrounded by an amorphous ground substance of structural glycoproteins—mainly fibronectin, laminin, and proteogylcans rich in sulfated heparin—reinforced by reticulin fibers. The lamina recticularis, containing fibronectin, is synthesized by and continuous with the underlying connective tissue. The BM serves as a tissue boundary to which cells attach and as a filter with selective permeability. The BM varies in thickness from site to site; most BMs are 15 to 50 nm thick, but the normal glomerular basement membrane (GBM) may be up to 350 nm thick.[1,2]

In most tissues, the BM is difficult to discern with the hematoxylin and eosin stain. Two methods are commonly used for demonstration of the BM: the periodic acid–methenamine silver (PAMS) and periodic acid–Schiff (PAS) methods. In both methods, the principle of oxidation-reduction, also referred to as an oxidation-aldehyde demonstration technique, is employed. The oxidation-reduction technique includes (1) the oxidation of carbohydrates to aldehyde groups with the use of an oxidizer, such as periodic acid or chromic acid; (2) binding of the stain to the newly formed aldehyde groups; (3) reduction and visualization of the binding site; and (4) final removal of the remaining stain. The oxidation step is controlled by time, with subsequent rinsing to remove excess acid.[3]

In the PAMS method, the newly created aldehydes have argentaffinic activity and will reduce methenamine silver solution to metallic silver. The metallic silver is replaced by gold in the toning reaction using gold chloride. All remaining unreduced silver and gold are removed with sodium thiosulfate. Methenamine silver staining is a progressive process; the end point must be closely monitored. The longer the slides are exposed to the silver solution, the more likely it is that overstaining will occur, often obscuring the fine details needed to properly assess the glomerular BMs, an essential element in the diagnosis of renal disease. This technique will stain all BMs in the kidney (glomerular, tubular, and Bowman's capsule), as well as the reticulin components. Silver impregnates only the lamina densa of the GBM and does not stain immunoglobulin deposits.[4]

In the PAS reaction, carbohydrates containing neutral hexose sugars and/or sialic acid are oxidized with periodic acid to form aldehydes. This step is followed by treatment with Schiff reagent (a solution of basic fuchsin reduced to a colorless compound by treatment with sulfurous acid), which binds to the newly formed aldehydes. A subsequent wash in running water results in loss of bound sulfurous acid groups and in visualization of the dye, which is typically magenta. A final rinse in metabisulfite removes excess Schiff reagent, and a counterstain is applied to demonstrate other tissue structures.[5]

Controls

A section of kidney containing both cortex and medulla serves as an appropriate control. Sections of the patient's tissue and the control tissue should be cut at 2 to 3 μm; thicker sections are not appropriate. The use of the microscope and knowledge of the microscopic appearance of the tissue is critical when determining the end point of the silver reaction. Renal tissue is extremely sensitive to the PAS reaction and quickly indicates depleted, overused, or inferior reagents.[5]

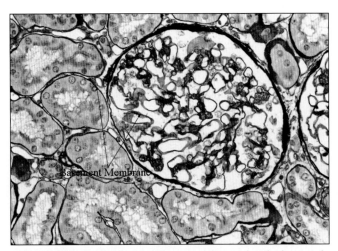

Figure 13.1. This section of kidney is well stained with the periodic acid–methenamine silver (PAMS) technique. The glomerular basement membrane appears as a fine, continuous, black line.

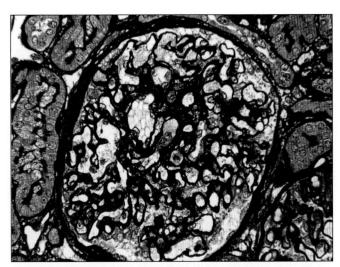

Figure 13.3. The glomerular basement membrane in this section of renal tissue is overstained. The silver is too dark, obscuring the fine details.

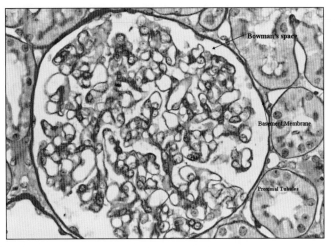

Figure 13.2. The glomerular basement membrane is stained magenta in this periodic acid–Schiff technique.

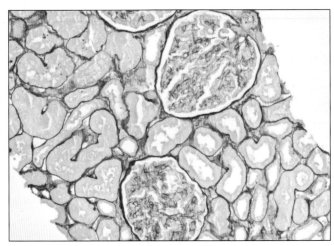

Figure 13.4. The glomerular basement membrane in this section is too light. The tissue section was not stained long enough. The mesangium, the basement membrane of Bowman's capsule, and the renal tubules can be identified, but not the capillary loops in the glomerulus.

What Should Be Seen in a Good Basement Membrane Stain

In the normal kidney, a typical glomerulus contains six to eight lobules composed of capillary loops and centrally located mesangium.[6] With both PAMS (Figure 13.1) and PAS (Figure 13.2), the BM of the loops should appear as a fine continuous line. The BM of the renal tubules should not be considered when determining the quality of the stain.[5,7]

Problems Encountered With the Methenamine Silver Reaction

PROBLEM: Determining the End Point of the Reaction

APPEARANCE: Overstaining obscures the fine details of the GBMs. The GBM is densely stained and may be either dark brown or black (Figure 13.3). With understained GBMs, the fine details may not be visible or the GBM may be light violet (Figure 13.4).

CAUSES:

- Reagents were improperly prepared and/or stored.
- Sections were removed from the heated silver solution too soon or too late.
- Old or "exhausted" reagents were used.

SOLUTIONS:

- Carefully check the preparation of the solutions, including percentages.
- Microscopically evaluate the end point of the stain. Look for the tan-brown color that develops, and stop the reaction when the appropriate structures can be identified microscopically.
- Evaluate only the GBM in determining the end point; ignore the renal tubular BM.

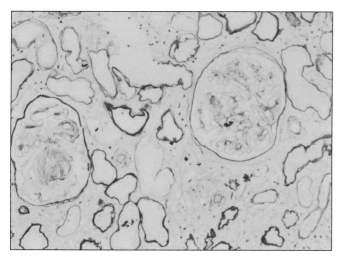

Figure 13.5. Nonspecific staining appears throughout this section.

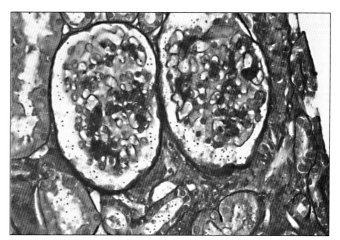

Figure 13.6. This slide, stained on an automated stainer, demonstrates precipitate and nonspecific staining.

- Ensure that only fresh solutions are used.
- Keep the silver solution and all reagents used to prepare the silver solution refrigerated.

COMMENTS: Experience in looking at slides microscopically during the staining process is invaluable in determining the end point of the reaction. If sections are overstained, obscuring many of the tissue components, remove excess silver by dipping the slide quickly in a very dilute solution of potassium ferricyanide.[7] Old or overused silver solutions may pose a safety hazard.[8]

PROBLEM: Nonspecific Staining of Tissue Elements, or Precipitate on Tissue, or Both

APPEARANCE: Tiny black granules appear on and around the tissue. Tissue components other than BMs are stained black (Figures 13.5 and 13.6). The background of the slide may have a blackish silver coloration, resembling a mirror (Figure 13.7).

CAUSES:
- The silver solution was overheated.
- The glassware was not cleaned properly.
- Metal instruments were used during the staining process.
- Overstaining occurred in the silver solution.

SOLUTIONS:
- Use clean, chemically treated glassware; chemical cleaners include concentrated nitric acid, bleach, and commercial glass cleaner.
- Use freshly prepared solutions.
- Use plastic holders or forceps when transferring slides between solutions.
- Microscopically determine the end point for the silver stain.

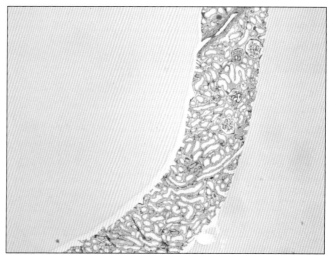

Figure 13.7. Mirroring appears on this slide, due to breakdown of the methenamine silver solution.

COMMENTS: Silver solutions degrade very rapidly when heated. Solutions should be fresh; make only a small quantity. Impeccably cleaned glassware is essential. Never use metal instruments in solution preparation and slide handling. Heat is an important factor when using methenamine silver, because the reaction time is accelerated with higher temperatures. Methenamine silver breaks down at temperatures in excess of 50°C, resulting in a mirrorlike deposition of silver on the inside of the Coplin jar and on the slide. The methenamine hydrolyzes at high temperatures, forming ammonia and formaldehyde. Formaldehyde reacts with the silver, reducing it to a metallic state.[9]

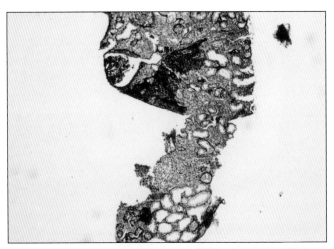

Figure 13.8. This tissue section is detaching and folding back upon itself, obscuring diagnostic tissue elements.

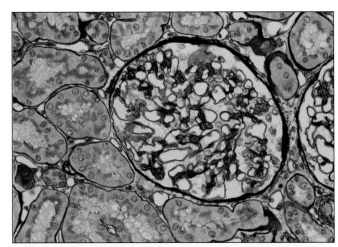

Figure 13.9. All tissue structures in this figure have a grayish appearance, and there is uneven staining.

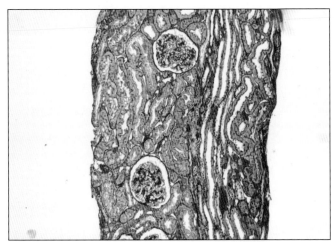

Figure 13.10. This slide was stained on an automated stainer. It appears that a reagent was not properly applied or that rinsing was not adequate to remove residual stains. This section has a golden hue on one edge of the tissue, while appearing normal on the remainder of the section.

PROBLEM: Difficulty in Keeping the Tissue Section on the Slide

APPEARANCE: All or part of the tissue section is missing from the slide (Figure 13.8).

CAUSES:

- When heated, methenamine breaks down into formaldehyde and ammonia. Because it is a strong base, ammonia can cause the tissue to detach from the slide because of the increased pH. Borax (sodium borate) used in the working solution controls the pH.

- Noncharged slides or excessive water bath adhesive were used during microtomy.

- Slides were not dried properly; water was not removed from under the tissue section.

SOLUTIONS:

- Properly drain and dry slides before staining.
- Use "plus" or positively charged slides.
- Ensure that the borax solution is fresh.
- Check the pH of the staining solutions (the pH should be 8.2).
- Do not overheat the solutions.
- Check the temperature of the slide-drying oven (approximately 60°C).

COMMENTS: It is a good practice to monitor the pH of the solutions used in the procedure. Using charged slides for all silver stains decreases the possibility of tissue detachment.

PROBLEM: Uneven Staining

APPEARANCE: The tissue may have an overall grayish appearance (Figure 13.9). If a microwave is used to accelerate the reaction, sections at the bottom of the slide may be more lightly stained than sections at the top (Figure 13.10).

CAUSES:

- There is inadequate or excessive heating of the silver solution.

- If a microwave oven is used, the temperature may be too high for proper staining; solutions should be approximately 95°C degrees when removed from the microwave.

- The temperature of the slides decreases during microscopic evaluation.

SOLUTIONS:

- When checking slides microscopically for end results, ensure that the slides are rinsed in 70°C distilled water before and after observation.

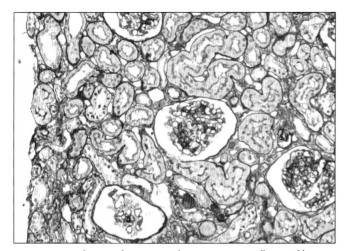

Figure 13.11. This tissue has a grey-violet appearance, usually caused by over-toning in gold chloride.

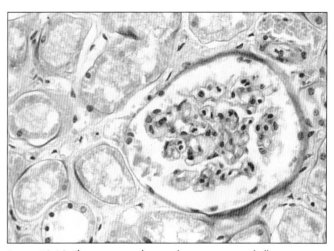

Figure 13.12. This section is understained; staining is not as brilliant as expected when using fresh Schiff reagent.

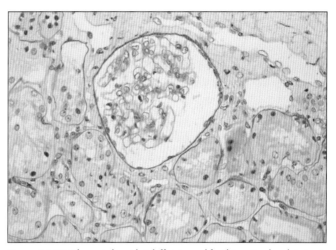

Figure 13.13. The periodic acid–Schiff stain used for this section has deteriorated; the tissue elements are pale pink.

- Monitor the temperature of the reagents used in the stain; this practice is particularly important when using a microwave-accelerated protocol.

COMMENTS: The use of a microwave oven to accelerate the staining reaction may magnify problems caused by inadequate washing of the slides after oxidation or the use of inadequately cleaned glassware.[3]

PROBLEM: Sections Overtoned in Gold Chloride

APPEARANCE: The tissue has a nonspecific, grey-violet coloration (Figure 13.11).

CAUSE:

- The slides are toned too long in gold chloride.

SOLUTIONS:

- Place slides in 3% sodium metabisulfite for 1 to 3 minutes.
- Check slides microscopically throughout the staining process.
- Carefully monitor the time that the slides are left in the gold chloride solution.

Problems Encountered With the Periodic Acid–Schiff Reaction

PROBLEM: Reaction Not as Bright as Expected; GBMs Not Stained Adequately

APPEARANCE: Instead of the brilliant magenta typically observed, the positive tissue components are stained pale pink (Figures 13.12 and 13.13).

CAUSES:

- Deteriorated or expired Schiff reagent was used.
- Schiff reagent was overused.
- The time in each solution was not adequately monitored.

- The strength of the periodic acid solution is incorrect.

SOLUTIONS:

- Use fresh Schiff reagent. Check the expiration date.
- Keep Schiff reagent refrigerated.
- Pink-tinged Schiff reagent may indicate overuse.
- Replace the periodic acid with a fresh 0.5% to 1.0% solution.
- Check slides microscopically to determine the end point of the stain.

COMMENTS: Although some solutions may be used beyond the expiration date, a test control section should be stained and compared to a prior control section to determine the adequacy of the stain.[2] The importance of running controls to determine optimal staining before using any reagents on the patient tissue cannot be overemphasized. Schiff reagent should be colorless or straw colored. To test Schiff reactivity, add 1 to 2 drops of

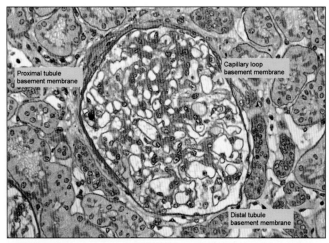

Figure 13.14. Tissue elements have a diffuse pink-red appearance, making specific tissue components difficult to visualize.

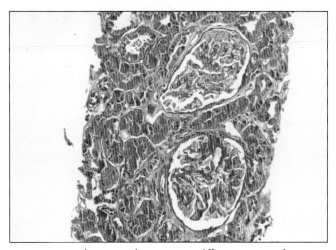

Figure 13.15. This section demonstrates a different intensity of magenta. Although tissue elements are visible, the fine details of the glomerular basement membrane are not distinct.

Schiff reagent to 10 mL of 37% formaldehyde. If the solution rapidly turns reddish purple, the reagent is still usable. If the reaction is delayed or the color is deep blue-purple, the solution has reached its end point and should be discarded.[5,7]

PROBLEM: Nonspecific Background Staining

APPEARANCE: Every tissue component appears to be staining to some degree with the Schiff reagent (Figures 13.14 and 13.15).

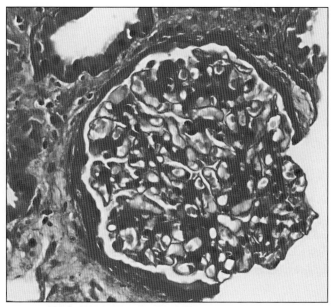

Figure 13.16. The hematoxylin counterstain has masked the positive Schiff staining on this slide.

CAUSES:

- Carryover of reagents has occurred at one or more steps of the process.
- Deteriorated Schiff reagent was used.
- If the periodic acid is not removed sufficiently, the aldehyde groups may overstain with the Schiff reagent.
- If the Schiff reagent is not completely removed, nonspecific adsorption can occur on the tissue.

SOLUTIONS:

- Wash sections thoroughly between each step in the procedure.
- Perform a viability check of the Schiff reagent.

COMMENTS: It is important to adhere to the times indicated. Stains should be optimized before use on a patient's material. Adequate washing is very important for the removal of solutions used in previous steps.

PROBLEM: Schiff Reaction Masked by Counterstain

APPEARANCE: The blue hematoxylin counterstain is too intense and masks the magenta-red color of the Schiff reaction. The contrast needed to adequately assess the GBM may be compromised (Figures 13.16 and 13.17).

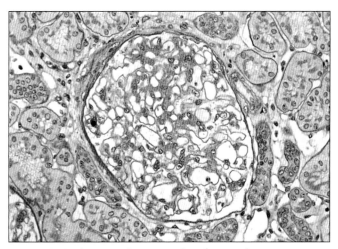

Figure 13.17. This section demonstrates loss of contrast between tissue structures, due to excessive counterstaining.

CAUSE:

- Sections were in hematoxylin counterstain too long.

SOLUTIONS:

- Control the time for the counterstain step in the procedure; in an optimal stain, the delicate blue nuclear stain is well balanced against the bright magenta-stained tissue components.

- Use a progressive type of hematoxylin or a diluted hematoxylin for counterstaining.

References

1. Bancroft JD, Gamble M. *Theory and Practice of Histological Techniques.* 5th ed. New York, NY: Churchill Livingstone; 1996: 139-144.

2. Jenis EH, Lowenthal DT. *Kidney Biopsy Interpretation.* 2nd ed. Philadelphia, PA: FA Davis Company; 1978: 1-10.

3. Grizzle WE. Theory and practice of silver staining in histopathology. *J Histotechnol.* 1996;19:183-194.

4. Ferrera GA, Lott RL. Silver stains in diagnostic renal pathology. *J Histotechnol.* 1996;19:219-223.

5. Carson, FL. *Histotechnology: A Self-Instructional Text.* 2nd ed. Chicago, IL: American Society of Clinical Pathologists; 1997: 113, 114, 149-150.

6. Wheater PR, Burkett HG, Daniels VG. *Functional Histology: A Text and Colour Atlas.* New York, NY: Churchill Livingstone; 1979: 49-56.

7. Sheehan DC, Hrapchak BB. *Theory and Practice of Histotechnology.* St Louis, MO: CV Mosby; 1980: 181-188, 352.

8. Titford M. Safety considerations in the use of silver stains. *J Histotechnol.* 1996;19:197-202

8. Churukian CJ. Consistent silver methods for demonstrating basement membranes, reticulum and fungi. *J Histotechnol.* 1996;19:211-217.

Mucin Stains

Freida L. Carson

Mucin is a term that is applied to a variety of cellular secretions, which are also known as mucopolysaccharides, mucosubstances, and glycoproteins. Cells from different parts of the body secrete slightly different mucins that may look similar macroscopically and microscopically, but they differ histochemically and are usually classified as either acidic or neutral mucins. The acidic mucins are further classified according to whether they are sulphated ($-OSO_3H$) and/or carboxylated ($-COOH$). Acidic mucins are found in connective tissue and in most mucin-secreting epithelial cells, whereas neutral mucin is abundant in Brunner glands and in the gastric foveolar epithelial cells. Neutral mucin is also present to some degree in goblet cells of the gastrointestinal and respiratory tracts and in the prostatic glands. Although mucin can be demonstrated by a variety of techniques, the most frequently used are Mayer mucicarmine, Alcian blue, and periodic acid–Schiff, with colloidal iron occasionally used.

Perhaps the most common technique for demonstrating acidic mucins is Mayer mucicarmine. This is an empirical stain, but it is thought that the aluminum forms a chelation complex with the carmine, resulting in a positively charged compound, which then attaches to the acidic, or negatively charged, groups (sulfate and/or carboxylate) of mucin. According to Horobin and Bancroft,[1] carmine is an ill-defined extract of the cochineal beetle, with carminic acid as the active constituent. They state that the chelate formed with aluminum is probably a cationic 2:1 carminic acid:aluminum complex. The selectivity of the stain for mucin, without displacing the hematoxylin from the previously stained nuclei, is probably due to the large size of the dye, resulting in a slow rate of dye diffusion and therefore restriction to the permeable and rapidly stained mucin. In a study by Laurén and Sorvari,[2] the specificity of the mucicarmine stain was compared to eight other techniques for mucin, and the staining pattern was observed to be comparable with that of Alcian blue.

Alcian blue is probably the most versatile of the mucin-staining techniques. It is a water-soluble, copper phthalocyanin basic dye, most commonly used in a 3% acetic acid solution, with a resulting pH of 2.5. Alcian blue is believed to form ionic bonds with the acidic groups (sulfate and/or carboxylate) of mucin. When it becomes diagnostically significant to distinguish whether a mixture of carboxyl and sulfate groups or only sulfate groups are present, selective staining of these tissue components is readily accomplished by Alcian blue. At a pH of 2.5, it will bind with both carboxyl and sulphated-ester groups, but if the pH is lowered to 1.0, Alcian blue will stain only sulfated mucins. Carboxyl groups are not ionized at the lower pH and therefore will not electrostatically attract the positively charged Alcian blue dye. Alcian blue with hyaluronidase was commonly used in the past to differentiate connective tissue mucin from epithelial mucin. At a pH of 2.5, Alcian blue with hyaluronidase digestion greatly reduces connective tissue mucin, while epithelial mucin is unaffected. Other than in combination with the periodic acid–Schiff (PAS) technique, the many other available variations of Alcian blue staining are not routinely used in the clinical laboratory. One of the advantages of Alcian blue over most of the other cationic dyes is that water, alcohol, weak acids, or counterstaining solutions will not extract it from stained sections. The incubation time for Alcian blue can be adjusted to achieve the desired results, with longer incubation times resulting in darker staining.

The PAS technique is also used to demonstrate mucins, and it is the only method that will demonstrate neutral mucins, such as that in the gastric foveolar epithelial cells. Some acidic mucins will also stain with the PAS technique. The PAS reaction is based on the oxidation by periodic acid of certain tissue groups, most commonly 1,2 glycols, to aldehydes. Schiff reagent is prepared by treating a solution of basic fuchsin with sulfurous acid, resulting in a reduced, colorless solution of

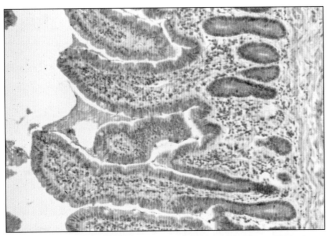

Figure 14.1. A good mucicarmine stain is illustrated in this figure. The mucin is well demonstrated, and both the iron hematoxylin and metanil yellow counterstains enhance the mucin staining.

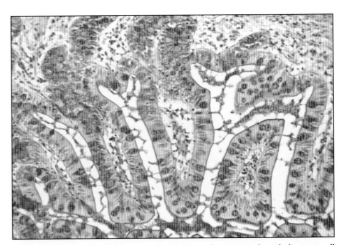

Figure 14.3. In this figure, mucin present in the intestinal epithelium is well demonstrated by a periodic acid–Schiff stain. The hematoxylin counterstain provides good contrast and does not mask the mucin staining.

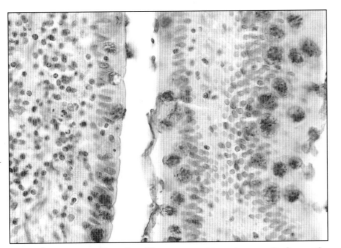

Figure 14.2. An excellent Alcian blue stain, pH 2.5, is shown in this figure. The mucin is very well demonstrated, and the nuclear fast red counterstain provides good contrast with the Alcian blue.

Although the exact mechanism of the reaction is not known, it is probable that the ferric ions form ionic bonds with the carboxyl groups of the acidic mucosubstances. The bound ferric iron is then demonstrated with the Prussian blue reaction. The color produced by this reaction is a much deeper, more intense shade of blue than that obtained with Alcian blue; however, colloidal iron is not as specific as Alcian blue for the acidic mucins. Strongly acidic mucins that do not stain with Alcian blue also will not stain with colloidal iron. This stain can also be combined with the PAS stain or with hyaluronidase digestion. Colloidal iron is an excellent method for the demonstration of *Cryptococcus neoformans*.

Controls

Sections from the gastrointestinal tract are most often used as mucin controls. The stomach contains primarily neutral mucin; therefore, it should not be used as a control for any mucin stain other than the PAS technique. Any section from the small intestine, colon, or appendix that is not autolyzed will be an excellent control for acidic mucins. The duodenum provides an excellent control if a combined Alcian blue-PAS stain is used, because the Brunner glands will stain only with the PAS reagent, and the goblet cells will show mixed Alcian blue and PAS staining. When the PAS stain is used, a small section of kidney should be included on the slide because it provides the most sensitive control for the viability of the reagents. When mucin stains are used for the diagnosis of adenocarcinoma, the control section should contain that tumor.

basic fuchsin, which then reacts with the aldehyde groups formed by periodic acid oxidation. Washing the slides in running water after the Schiff reaction will cause the loss of bound sulfurous acid, and the typical Schiff rose color results. If metabisulfite rinses are not used after the Schiff reaction, then copious running water must be used; otherwise, false colorization of some tissue elements will occur because of oxidation of adsorbed reagent.

Colloidal iron can also be used to demonstrate acidic mucins, because these mucins are the principle substances in tissues that will absorb colloidal ferric ions.

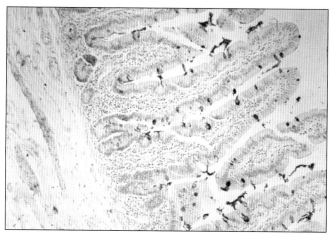

Figure 14.4. Acidic mucins are demonstrated with this colloidal iron stain. The mucin usually stains more intensely with colloidal iron than with Alcian blue, but the stain is not quite as specific.

What Should Be Seen in a Good Stain for Mucin

Regardless of the technique used, the mucin should be well stained and the counterstain should enhance the mucin staining. The contrast between the mucin and the other tissue components should be excellent, and no stain artifacts should be present. Good mucin stains by the various techniques are demonstrated in Figures 14.1 through 14.4.

Problems Encountered With the Mucicarmine Stain

PROBLEM: Weak Staining of Mucin

APPEARANCE: Mucin staining is weak and does not contrast well with the counterstain (Figures 14.5 and 14.6).

CAUSES:

- Mucicarmine solution has deteriorated. If the solution is prepared in-house, the carmine powder may not be of good composition.
- Stock solution has been stored at room temperature.

SOLUTIONS:

- Discard mucicarmine solution, and open or prepare a new stock solution.
- Prepare a new solution from a different carmine powder source.
- Discard stock solution, open or prepare a new stock solution, and keep it refrigerated.

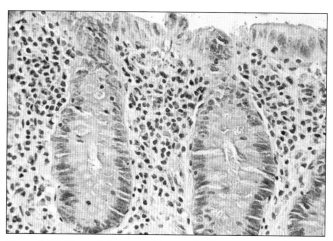

Figure 14.5. The mucin is very weakly stained with mucicarmine in this section of colon. The section has been counterstained with Weigert hematoxylin and metanil yellow.

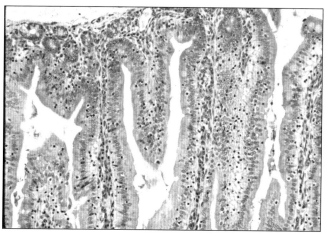

Figure 14.6. This section of small intestine illustrates goblet cells that are very weakly stained with mucicarmine. The counterstain is an aluminum hematoxylin.

COMMENTS: Mucicarmine stock stain solution deteriorates on standing, even with refrigeration, and should not be used for more than a few months. Commercial samples of carmine powder vary in composition and contain only 20% to 40% of the staining component,[1] so if the staining is weak with a new lot of powder, discard it and order new powder.

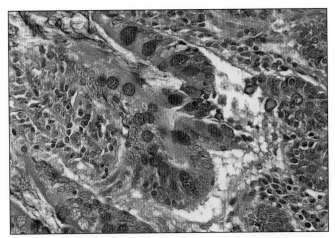

Figure 14.7. The metanil yellow counterstain is too intense in this section, decreasing the contrast between the mucicarmine-stained goblet cells and the background.

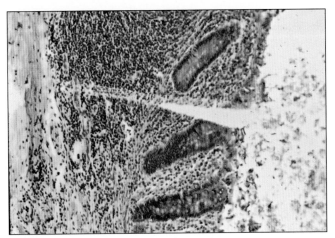

Figure 14.8. This low-magnification image of large intestine stained with mucicarmine illustrates the loss of contrast observed with excessive metanil yellow staining.

PROBLEM: Poor Counterstaining

APPEARANCE: The carminophilic properties of mucin are decreased, obscured, or masked by the counterstain (Figures 14.7 and 14.8).

CAUSES:

- There is overstaining with iron hematoxylin.
- There is overstaining with metanil yellow.

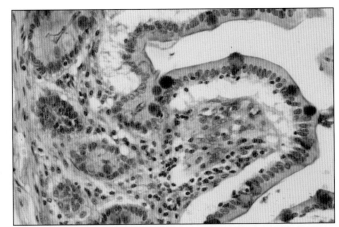

Figure 14.9. In this section of intestinal tract stained with Alcian blue, the background staining is very intense, with the connective tissue, nuclei, and goblet cells appearing almost the same shade of blue.

SOLUTIONS:

- Reduce staining time in iron hematoxylin solution.
- Reduce staining time in metanil yellow.

COMMENTS: Counterstaining with iron hematoxylin, aluminum hematoxylin, or metanil yellow should not be very intense. Although older texts specify that the Weigert hematoxylin should be made fresh, this solution will stain well for several days. Some hematoxylins, such as Ehrlich's, have been reported to add a bluish cast to the mucin.[1]

Problems Encountered With the Alcian Blue Stain

PROBLEM: Excessive Background Staining With Alcian Blue

APPEARANCE: The background tissues are excessively stained with Alcian blue. Although slight staining of the background connective tissue is normal, because of the content of acidic mucosubstances, it should not be very noticeable and should not detract from the specific mucin staining (Figures 14.9 and 14.10).

CAUSES:

- The pH is above 2.5.
- The dye might contain either salt or dextrin impurities.
- The staining time is too long.

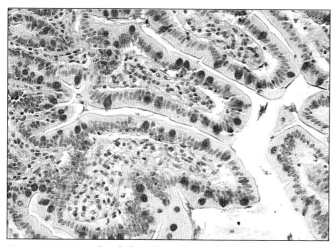

Figure 14.10. Even though the goblet cells are well stained, there is excessive staining of the connective tissue in this section of small intestine stained with Alcian blue. (Compare Figures 14.9 and 14.10 with Figure 14.2.)

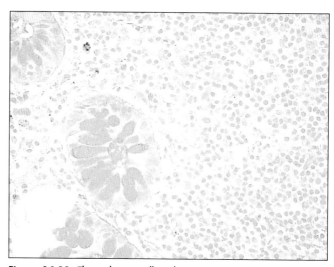

Figure 14.11. The nuclei, as well as the mucin, appear blue in this section stained with Alcian blue.

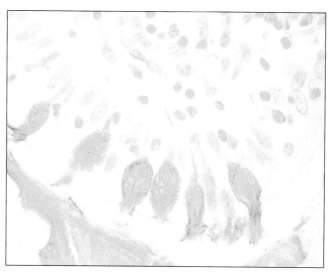

- The Alcian blue solution is too concentrated.
- Sections are not rinsed with acetic acid after staining with Alcian blue.

SOLUTIONS:
- Ensure that the staining solution is at the correct pH.
- Discard the dye and obtain a new batch.
- Vary the staining time.
- Decrease the dye concentration. Both the staining time and the dye concentration may have to be varied with different dye lots.
- Rinse sections with 3% acetic acid after the Alcian blue staining to prevent nonspecific staining.

PROBLEM: Nuclei Stained With Alcian Blue

APPEARANCE: The nuclei are stained with Alcian blue (Figures 14.11 and 14.12).

CAUSES:
- Staining was prolonged in Alcian blue.
- There was improper rinsing after the Alcian blue stain.

SOLUTIONS:
- Shorten the staining time in Alcian blue.
- Rinse with 3% acetic acid after the Alcian blue stain.

Figure 14.12. A high-magnification image of the same Alcian-blue–stained section seen in Figure 14.11, demonstrating the blue-stained chromatin of the nuclei.

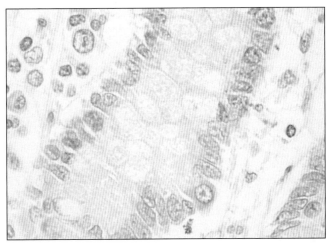

Figure 14.13. The goblet cells are very weakly stained with Alcian blue in this figure. (Compare the staining with that seen in Figure 14.2, an excellent Alcian blue stain.)

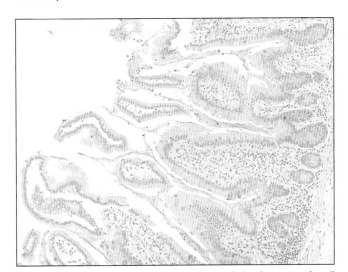

Figure 14.14. Although the goblet cells can be identified in this section of small intestine, they are poorly stained with Alcian blue. (Compare with the intensity of an excellent Alcian blue stain, as seen in Figure 14.2.)

PROBLEM: Weak Alcian Blue Staining in Structures Expected to be Positive

APPEARANCE: Structures expected to be positive (ie, goblet cells) are only weakly stained with Alcian blue (Figures 14.13, 14.14, and 14.15).

CAUSES:

- The dye solution was weak.
- There was poor hydration during deparaffinization steps.

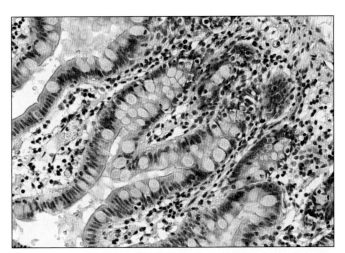

Figure 14.15. The goblet cells are poorly stained in this section of intestine stained with Alcian blue. The contrast provided by the hematoxylin counterstain is not as good as that of nuclear fast red.

SOLUTIONS:

- Discard dye or solution and obtain a new batch. The Alcian blue may not have completely dissolved or may have precipitated from solution. Do not use Alcian blue 5G or 7G; Alcian blue 8GX is the best dye for this technique. If 8GX is not available, use 8GS.
- Extend the hydration step during deparaffinization, because some alcianophilic structures hydrate slowly.

Problems Encountered With the Periodic Acid–Schiff Stain

PROBLEM: Weak Staining

APPEARANCE: Structures expected to stain PAS positive are only weakly positive.

CAUSES:

- Schiff reagent is old or depleted.
- The periodic acid is of incorrect strength or has been misused.

SOLUTIONS:

- Schiff reagent should not be overused (this can easily happen).
- Store Schiff reagent in the refrigerator and use only colorless or straw-colored solution.
- Do not use the periodic acid repeatedly; for best results, it should be used for only one run and then discarded.

COMMENTS: Kidney tissue is the most sensitive control for the PAS reaction and quickly indicates depleted, overused, or inferior reagents[3] (Figures 14.16, 4,17, and 14.18). It is helpful to put a small piece of kidney tissue on control slides as well as the specific tissue for mucin.

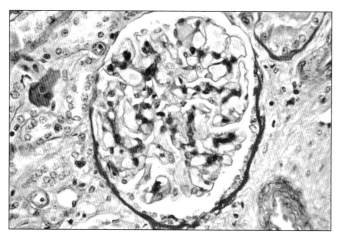

Figure 14.16. This section of kidney is an example of a good periodic acid–Schiff stain.

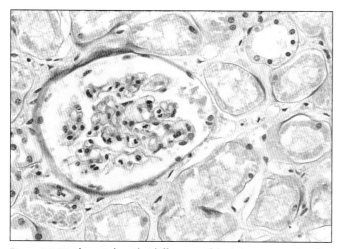

Figure 14.17. The periodic acid–Schiff staining of this kidney section is less than optimal, most likely due to overuse of the Schiff reagent. The mesangium and basement membranes show incomplete staining.

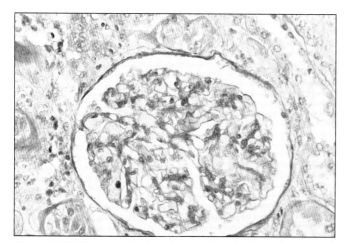

Figure 14.18. This section of kidney shows greatly reduced periodic acid–Schiff staining because of nonviable Schiff reagent.

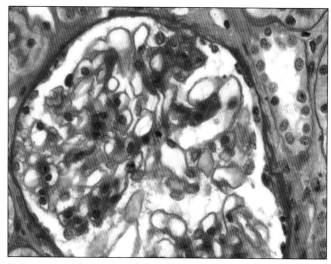

Figure 14.19. This section of kidney illustrates excessive background staining by the periodic acid–Schiff reaction.

PROBLEM: Staining of Unexpected Structures or Excessive Background Staining

APPEARANCE: There is excessive pink-rose Schiff staining of the background (Figure 14.19).

CAUSES:

- Schiff reagent may be old.
- There was carryover of the periodic acid.
- Artifactual aldehyde groups may be present because of glutaraldehyde fixation or insufficient washing of tissue after formaldehyde fixation.
- There was insufficient removal of the Schiff reagent, allowing nonspecific adsorption on the tissue.

SOLUTIONS:

- Discard Schiff reagent and use fresh solution.
- Rinse sections well after periodic acid oxidation.
- Rinse sections well after formaldehyde fixation; the problem with glutaraldehyde fixation cannot be corrected.
- Rinse sections thoroughly before staining with the Schiff reagent.

COMMENTS: Although many procedures omit the metabisulfite rinses after the Schiff reagent, several prominent histochemists consider the sulfite rinses essential to remove any uncombined leucofuchsin after exposure to the Schiff reagent.[3] Sections can be oxidized by highly chlorinated tap water. If sections are transferred from the Schiff reagent immediately into tap water, any loosely adsorbed Schiff reagent may be reoxidized to basic fuchsin, which may then nonspecifically stain the tissue. The metabisulfite rinses must be followed by running water. If they are omitted, then a rapid and copious running water wash must be used after the Schiff reagent.

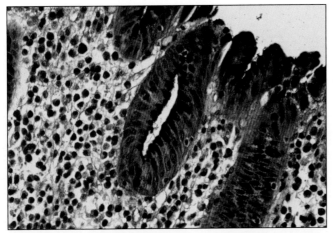

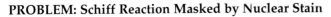

Figure 14.20. This periodic acid-Schiff–stained section of intestinal tract demonstrates marked overstaining with hematoxylin. No chromatin patterns can be seen in the very densely stained nuclei, and the hematoxylin masks much of the Schiff reaction.

PROBLEM: Schiff Reaction Masked by Nuclear Stain

APPEARANCE: The counterstain (hematoxylin) is much too dark, masking the Schiff reaction (Figure 14.20).

CAUSE:

• Staining was prolonged in the hematoxylin solution.

SOLUTION:

• Decrease the staining time in hematoxylin.

Problems Encountered With the Colloidal Iron Stain

PROBLEM: Marked Background Staining

APPEARANCE: Marked staining of the connective tissue (Figures 14.21 and 14.22). Some staining is normal, but it should be very light.

CAUSES:

• Old solutions were used.
• Acidified rinses were not performed, the colloidal iron solution was not acidified,[4] or both.

SOLUTIONS:

• Prepare fresh colloidal iron solution, including the use of fresh solutions in the preparation of this reagent.
• Ensure that the colloidal iron solution is acidified, and use 12% acetic acid rinses before and after the colloidal iron solution.

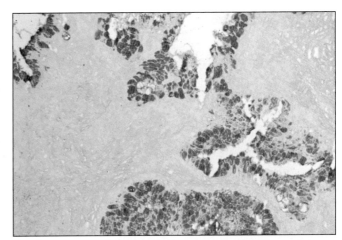

Figure 14.21. This section of cervix is stained with colloidal iron and demonstrates overstaining of the connective tissue mucins. No counterstain was used on this section.

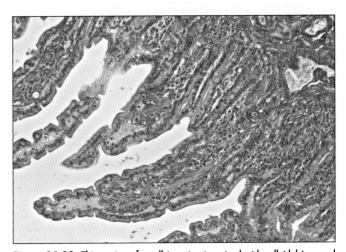

Figure 14.22. This section of small intestine is stained with colloidal iron and demonstrates marked nonspecific staining of the connective tissue. This stain should be repeated using freshly prepared solutions.

References

1. Horobin RW, Bancroft JD. *Troubleshooting Histology Stains.* New York, NY: Churchill Livingstone; 1998: 194-197.

2. Laurén PA, Sorvari TE. The histochemical specificity of mucicarmine staining in the identification of epithelial mucosubstances. *Acta Histochem.* 1969;34: 263-272.

3. Carson FL. *Histotechnology: A Self-Instructional Text.* 2nd ed. Chicago, IL: American Society of Clinical Pathologists; 1997: 113-114.

4. Sheehan DC, Hrapchak BB. *Theory and Practice of Histotechnology.* St. Louis, MO: CV Mosby; 1980: 171.

Amyloid

Vinnie Della Speranza

The term amyloid, meaning starch-like, is a misnomer coined by Virchow when he observed that amyloid deposits would stain blue with the iodine reaction, suggesting the presence of starch or cellulose. Despite a striking morphologic uniformity in virtually all cases, amyloid is now known to encompass a spectrum of secondary protein structure diseases.[1] The only common denominator is the tendency of these proteins, under specific circumstances, to form β-pleated sheets of antiparallel fibrils, regardless of the source protein's original primary structure or function.[2]

Amyloid deposits occur insidiously and may be found in many organs, often in the walls of small blood vessels. Definitive diagnosis requires the morphologic identification of amyloid deposits in biopsies of the affected organs, which may be surprisingly difficult. Amyloid deposits have a characteristic amorphous hyaline or glassy appearance, but otherwise they stain no differently from other proteins in a routine hematoxylin and eosin stain.

The progressive accumulation of extracellular protein fibrils can lead to cellular atrophy, ischemia, necrosis, and, ultimately, organ failure due to the detrimental effect of these accumulated fibrils on blood supply and normal cellular function; therefore, correct recognition of amyloid deposits is of considerable importance in diagnostic surgical pathology.[3] The clinician will have many questions for the pathologist: Is the amyloid systemic or localized? Is the amyloidosis primary, secondary, or inherited? The answers to these questions are important because patients with localized disease do not require systemic therapy, and their long-term prognosis is excellent. The prognosis and treatment modalities for the three forms of systemic amyloidosis differ significantly, making accurate characterization essential.[4]

All amyloid deposits share the following physical properties:

- Appearance of amorphous, eosinophilic deposits under light microscopy after hematoxylin and eosin staining
- Bright green birefringence under polarized light after staining with the cotton-wool dye Congo red

- Regular fibrillary structure observed with electron microscopy
- β-pleated-sheet structure demonstrated with x-ray diffraction[5]

By definition, any protein deposits staining with Congo red and exhibiting green birefringence when viewed with polarized light are amyloid.[4] Although the identification of amyloid deposits in tissues without characterization of the source protein is not especially helpful to the clinician, the use of tinctorial stains remains an important screening tool for the initial diagnosis of amyloidosis.

Other cotton dyes have been explored for amyloid staining with varying success, most notably Sirius red. This dye has failed to gain popularity, however, because it does not exhibit the polarizing characteristics considered the hallmark of amyloid staining with Congo red. The presence of carbohydrate moieties in amyloid fibrils has encouraged some investigators to use carbohydrate stains, such as periodic acid–Schiff or Alcian blue, to demonstrate amyloid deposits; however, dye uptake is variable and generally poor with these methods. Likewise, metachromatic stains, such as crystal violet or methyl violet, attempt to capitalize on the carbohydrate content of amyloid fibrils, but their staining is not very specific, and the low sensitivity of these methods has caused them to fall in disfavor.

Staining with fluorochrome thioflavin T is an alternate method to improve the sensitivity of amyloid detection; however, the stained sections are not permanent, and tissue components other than amyloid, including fibrinoid, keratin, intestinal muciphages, Paneth cells, zymogen granules, and juxtaglomerular apparatus, all stain with thioflavin T.[6] Furthermore, the appropriate excitation and barrier filters required for fluorescence microscopy may not be available in most laboratories. Therefore, Congo red, specifically the alkaline Congo red method of Puchtler et al,[7] remains the gold standard for the demonstration of amyloid in tissue sections.

With the Congo red stain, false-positive or false-negative results are usually related to (1) the staining technique, (2) the microscope equipment, or (3) the presence

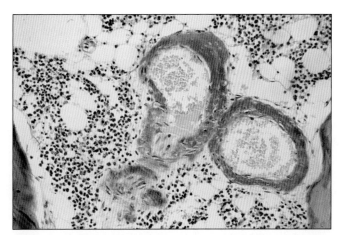

Figure 15.1. This bone marrow section stained with the Puchtler Congo red procedure reveals intense amyloid deposits in the bone marrow sample. (Photo courtesy of Freida Carson, PhD.)

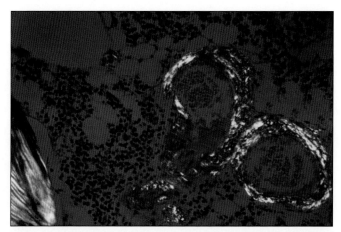

Figure 15.2. This figure shows the same section seen in Figure 15.1 but viewed with polarizing microscopy; amyloid deposits exhibit characteristic apple-green birefringence. (Photo courtesy of Freida Carson, PhD.)

of small amounts of amyloid.[2] Congo red in aqueous solution will bind nonspecifically to many tissue structures, including collagen and elastin. Excessive differentiation may lead to decolorization of the amyloid, while collagen remains stained. The Benhold Congo red technique does not yield reproducible results and should be avoided.[2]

The use of alcoholic solutions, high salt content, and high pH, as in the Puchtler Congo red method, greatly increase staining specificity for amyloid. A saturated salt solution in alcohol at alkaline pH is used in both the dye solution and as a pretreatment of the tissue sections just before staining. High salt content and alkaline pH are believed to depress dye ionization and electrostatic binding to nonamyloid structures. Saturation of the salt and dye solutions is very important, and the instructions must be followed exactly.[3]

The Congo red stain can be applied to tissues fixed in a variety of fixative solutions, including Bouin, Helly, Zenker, ethanol, and formalin; this technique is also effective for frozen sections and cytology smears. This versatility makes the Congo red stain suitable for the examination of tissues in many settings, including the examination of archival tissues in paraffin blocks. Tissues that have been stored for prolonged periods in formalin will have diminished staining; therefore, fixation for inordinately long periods should be avoided.[2,6] One report indicates that Carnoy fixative confers a greater risk of false-positive staining[8] and should be avoided.

Controls

Virtually any tissue containing known deposits of amyloid may be used as a suitable control. However, as previously stated, fixation for prolonged periods may diminish staining; therefore, tissues identified as positive for amyloid should be processed immediately into paraffin blocks. Large deposits of amyloid (presumably older deposits) frequently show less intense staining and may not exhibit green birefringence with polarized light.[9] Smaller deposits, thought to represent more recent amyloid deposits, can often be found in blood vessel walls and tend to make better controls.

One author has reported that sections that have been precut and stored will lose staining reactivity over time; therefore, it is recommended that control sections should be relatively freshly cut. Sections of 6- to 8-μm thickness are most desirable, because this thickness increases the likelihood of discovering small amyloid deposits. Thinner sections may fail to exhibit birefringence.[3]

What Should Be Seen in a Good Congo Red Stain

In a section that has been well stained with Congo red, the staining should be limited to amyloid deposits present in the tissue section. In general, amyloid will appear a muted red or pink color, the intensity of which is largely dependent upon the size, density, and age of the amyloid deposit (Figure 15.1).

The Congo red-stained section will also show green birefringence with polarizing microscopy; this finding is mandatory for diagnosing amyloid (Figure 15.2). It should be noted that other tissue elements, including collagen, smooth muscle, and striated muscle, will also display birefringence of varying colors that may be mistaken for amyloid.

Evaluation of Congo red-stained sections with a fluorescence microscope also may be used to identify minute amyloid deposits. Using a fluorescein isothiocyanate filter, amyloid deposits appear yellow-orange, increasing the sensitivity of the technique. However, Congo red fluorescence is not specific, and the presence of characteristic green birefringence with polarizing microscopy should be confirmed in deposits identified with fluorescence microscopy.[10]

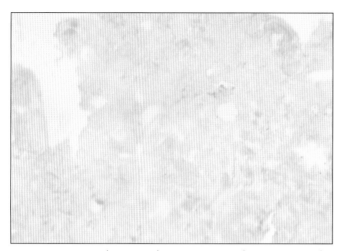

Figure 15.3. Congo red staining in this section appears indistinct, suggesting that the stain was excessively differentiated.

Problems Encountered With the Congo Red Stain

PROBLEM: Weakly Stained Tissues

APPEARANCE: Faint uptake of Congo red dye throughout the section (Figures 15.3 and 15.4).

CAUSES:

- Tissue was fixed for a prolonged period in a formaldehyde-containing fixative.
- Cut sections were stored for a prolonged period.
- Solutions of Congo red are not stable in the presence of salt and alkali.

SOLUTIONS:

- Avoid storing tissues in formaldehyde-based fixatives for prolonged periods of time.
- Cut the sections just before staining, or cut only as many control sections as can be used in a short period of time.
- Seal the cut paraffin blocks to help preserve control tissue reactivity.
- Prepare fresh working solutions just before use.[11]

PROBLEM: Nonspecific Staining

APPEARANCE: Structures other than amyloid bind the Congo red; high background staining may make it difficult to distinguish true amyloid deposits if present in the tissue (Figures 15.5 and 15.6).

CAUSES:

- Collagen, elastic fibers, and keratin may stain nonspecifically with some fixatives and some procedures.
- Aqueous Congo red solutions have a tendency to stain structures nonspecifically; this is especially true of the original Benhold formulation.
- The pH is not sufficiently alkaline.

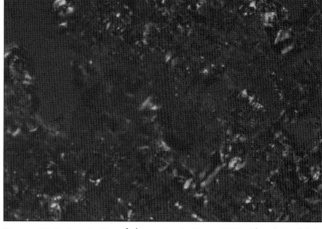

Figure 15.4. Examination of the section in Figure 15.3 with polarized light reveals numerous amyloid deposits.

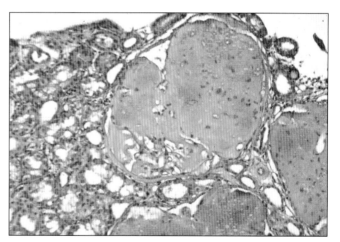

Figure 15.5. Tissue components in this Congo red-stained kidney section appear to be nonspecifically stained.

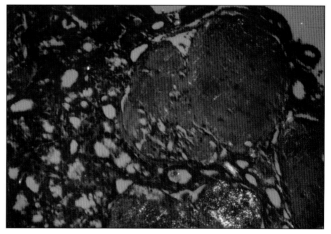

Figure 15.6. Polarization of the Congo red-stained section seen in Figure 15.5 reveals that most of the red staining is not amyloid. Some apple-green birefringence is noted in the glomerulus at the bottom of the image.

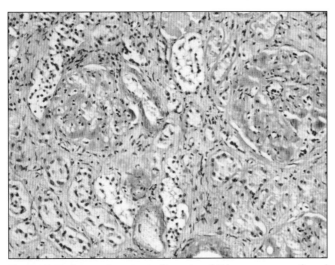

Figure 15.7. Congo red staining in this section of kidney appears specific and well differentiated.

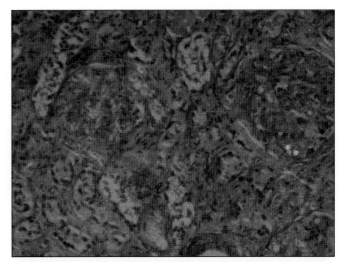

Figure 15.8. When viewed with polarized light, amyloid deposits seen in Figure 15.7 appear red to yellow, not the expected apple-green color; incorrect section thickness is the most likely cause.

SOLUTIONS:

- Use polarizing microscopy to help distinguish connective tissue components (grey or silver) from amyloid deposits (green).

- Rotating the slide on the stage during polarizing microscopy can help distinguish true amyloid deposits from connective tissue. When the slide is rotated, connective tissue fibers will lose the dichroism, while amyloid will not.[2]

- Use the Puchtler Congo red method, because the high salt content of the prestain rinse and staining solutions tends to diminish nonspecific staining.

- After staining, increase time in the alcoholic potassium hydroxide rinse to improve differentiation with the Highman technique.

- Avoid the use of Canada balsam mounting medium because it will fluoresce.[11]

PROBLEM: Incorrect Color of Birefringence

APPEARANCE: Structures may exhibit yellow, red, or white dichroism (Figures 15.7, 15.18, and 15.9).

CAUSE:

- Section thickness may be incorrect; this artifact is especially likely in thin sections.[3]

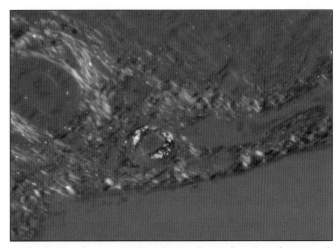

Figure 15.9. Collagen, appearing white to silver in this polarized, Congo red-stained section, surrounds a characteristic apple-green amyloid deposit.

SOLUTION:

- Ensure that sections are cut at 6 to 8 μm.

COMMENT: It should be noted that old (large) amyloid deposits will often display diminished birefringence. Smaller deposits in blood vessel walls, for example, may be more likely to demonstrate the characteristic apple-green color.

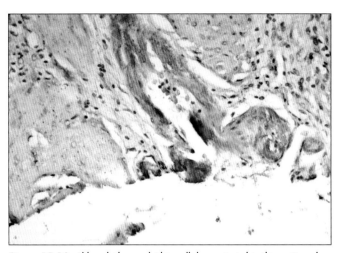

Figure 15.10. Although the amyloid is well demonstrated in this section, close inspection reveals a red granular precipitate caused by using isopropyl alcohol instead of ethyl alcohol as the solvent for the salt solutions. (Image courtesy of Janet Tunnicliffe, MLT, ART.)

PROBLEM: Precipitate on Tissue

APPEARANCE: A red precipitate is randomly present throughout the tissue (Figure 15.10).

CAUSE:

• Salt solutions were prepared with isopropyl alcohol.

SOLUTION:

• Ensure that the salt solutions are prepared with ethyl alcohol because the salt does not dissolve well in isopropyl alcohol and will deposit crystals on the section.

References

1. Kaplan B, Martin BM, Livneh A, Pras M, Gallo, GR. Biochemical subtyping of amyloid in formalin-fixed tissue samples confirms and supplements immuno-histologic data. *Am J Clin Pathol.* 2004;121:794-800.

2. Rocken C, Sletten K. Amyloid in surgical pathology. *Virchows Arch.* 2003;443:3-16.

3. Carson FL. *Histotechnology: A Self-Instructional Text.* 2nd ed. Chicago, IL: American Society of Clinical Pathologists; 1997: 125-129.

4. Gertz MA. The classification and typing of amyloid deposits. *Am J Clin Pathol.* 2004;121:787-789.

5. Baethge BA, Jacobson DR. Amyloidosis, overview. 2006 Aug 11. Available at: http://www.emedicine.com/med/topic3377.htm. Accessed November 12, 2008.

6. Bancroft JD, Gamble M. *Theory and Practice of Histological Techniques.* 5th ed. London, England: Churchill Livingstone; 2002: 303-320.

7. Sweat F, Levine M. On the binding of Congo red by amyloid. *J Histochem Cytochem.* 1962;10:355-364.

8. Carson FL, Kingsley WB. Nonamyloid green bire-fringence following Congo red staining. *Arch Pathol Lab Med.* 1980;104:333-335.

9. Geisinger KR, Stanley MW, Raab SS, Silverman JF, Abati A. *Modern Cytopathology.* London, England: Churchill Livingstone; 2004.

10. Fail M, Self S. A novel approach for the demonstration of amyloid in thin (2 micron) sections of kidney. *HistoLogic.* 2000;32:1-3.

11. Horobin RW, Bancroft JD. *Troubleshooting Histology Stains.* London, England: Churchill Livingstone; 2000.

Immunohistochemistry

Janet Tunnicliffe

Introduction

Since the mid-1980s, when immunohistochemistry (IHC) techniques started to move from research into the clinical laboratory, the basis of an antibody-antigen reaction complex has not changed. What has changed is the quality and availability of antibodies, the detection reagents, and the potential applications of the technique. These advances, combined with the use of best-practice techniques in the histology laboratory, have improved the reliability and reproducibility of IHC staining results to the level where IHC is now considered an essential part of the surgical consultation process.

Fixation

The role of a fixative is to stop the naturally occurring autolysis of cells upon removal from the body. Fixation is accomplished by the denaturing of cellular proteins via coagulation or the formation of additive compounds. Fixatives that preserve by coagulation (eg, alcohols) not only preserve the cellular structure, providing excellent cytoplasmic and nuclear detail, but cause less destruction of the epitope or antigen site on or in the cell. The main problem with coagulating fixatives is their poor penetration rate; therefore, coagulating fixatives are only suited to very small samples in which the fluid can completely penetrate the tissue in a short time. Formalin is the most common of the additive fixatives and, when applied in a buffered solution, provides morphologic preservation, rapid penetration, precise immunolocalization, and minimal masking of antigens. The formation of methylene bridges by formalin can block the epitope sites of some antigens, but with the use of improved methods of antigen retrieval, this problem has been almost eliminated, except in tissues that have been fixed for an extended period of time. The use of fixatives that contain heavy metals creates the same problems in IHC as in routine histology techniques, namely, disposal of the used fixative and the formation of precipitates in the tissue section. Use of approved handling, collection, and disposal methods should always be followed. The presence of precipitates is only a concern in that their chemical removal may negatively impact the antigenicity of

the tissue; therefore, if the precipitate does not interfere with the ability to interpret the IHC stain, the precipitate can remain in the section.

Antibody Selection and Use

Antibodies can be classified into two main categories, polyclonal and monoclonal, each with their own advantages and problems. Polyclonal antibodies are produced by multiple immune cells in the host animal after exposure to a single antigen. The result is an immune serum that contains more than one type of antibody, and thus the serum as a whole is capable of binding multiple epitopes, or binding sites, on the single antigen against which it was raised. Monoclonal antibodies are produced by a single clone of plasma cells, resulting in one type of antibody that will react only with a single, specific epitope on the antigen against which it was raised. Although monoclonal antibodies are highly specific, their efficacy can be greatly affected if the single epitope against which the antibody is directed is masked or destroyed during fixation or processing. In contrast, polyclonal antibodies may still be able to bind to one or more of the epitopes on the antigen that may have survived fixation and processing and are thus typically more sensitive. Antibodies can be purchased in many formats—ready to use, prediluted, concentrated, and lyophilized—each with inherent problems and advantages. The key to selecting the format is to remember that the goal of IHC is optimal specific staining with minimal nontarget staining. Development of an antibody-specific protocol allows the antibody dilution, method of antigen retrieval, incubation time, and incubation temperature to be controlled and reproduced for each specific antibody. When one or more of the parameters is preset, the user can only optimize the protocol by adjusting the remaining factors—a critical point to consider when selecting antibodies and or automated procedures.

Antigen Retrieval

The original antigen-unmasking techniques used proteolytic enzymes, such as trypsin, protease, or pepsin, with limited success. Enzymes can overdigest the coagulated

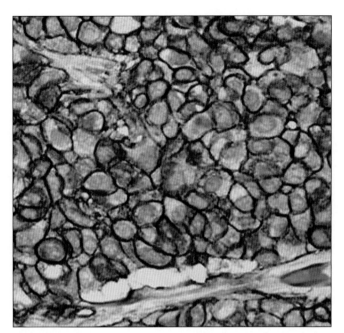

Figure 16.1. This breast cancer section is stained with a monoclonal antibody to HER 2 and demonstrates a cell membrane staining pattern.

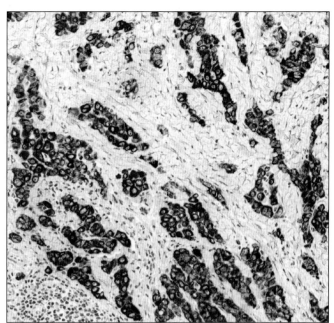

Figure 16.2. This invasive carcinoma section is stained with a cocktail of antibodies to cytokeratins and demonstrates a cytoplasmic staining pattern.

protein complexes, thereby reducing the overall antigen immunoreactivity. High enzyme concentration or extended exposure to enzymes can also cause severe tissue damage and loss of the section from the slide. Proteolytic enzymes applied according to strict protocols continue to be the optimal retrieval method for some antigens, such as cytokeratins. Heat-induced epitope retrieval (HIER), when first introduced, broke many preconceived boundaries. Heat was thought to denature protein and cause tissue damage, not unmask antigen binding sites. Although HIER is a well-recognized and documented procedure, there is little known about the physical chemistry of the HIER process, except that the damaging effects of heat are reduced with the use of buffered solutions such as tris(hydroxymethyl)-methylamine (TRIS), ethylenediaminetetraacetic acid (EDTA), or citrate in a range of pH 6 to 10. Again, the end user must test and validate an antigen-specific procedure that balances the type of antigen retrieval to be used, the strength or pH of the retrieval buffer, and the time of exposure to ensure the optimal IHC results.

Controls

All control material must be fixed, processed, and embedded in the same manner as the patient tissue to be tested. This protocol can be a challenge for larger facilities that receive requests from external sources. It is therefore critical that standard operating procedures (SOPs) be drafted and implemented with involvement of all stakeholders (submitting facilities) to ensure that the basic requirements—use of the correct fixative and duration of fixation and processing—are followed.

Controls for IHC can be divided into three major categories: negative controls, positive controls, and internal controls. The use of multi-tissue controls that combine negative and positive controls in a single paraffin block, sections of which are placed on each slide of the patient's specimen to be tested, is considered best practice.

Negative controls can be further subdivided into tissue negative controls and patient or reagent negative controls. Tissue negative controls are tissues that do not contain the target cell or antigen to which the antibody is directed. An example would be a slide of uterine tissue for a negative prostate-specific antigen (PSA) control. Any positive staining indicates either a technical error in the procedure or cross-reactivity of the antibody, and the result on the patient slide should be considered invalid. A patient or reagent negative control is a section of the patient tissue to be tested. This slide is stained following the identical protocol, except that the primary antibody is replaced with a nonreactive reagent, such as nonimmune sera, buffer, or antibody diluent. The expected result is that all cells should be negative; any positive staining indicates a cross-reaction between the patient tissue and the detection reagents or reaction with endogenous biotin in the patient tissue. Comparison of the patient negative control slide and the patient test slide will assist in the interpretation of any nonspecific background staining seen in the patient test slide.

Positive controls are essential for the validation of the antibody protocol and the continued testing of patient slides. Positive controls should be from several tissues with a range of antigenicity to assist in the selection of the correct dilution of the primary antibody. If only

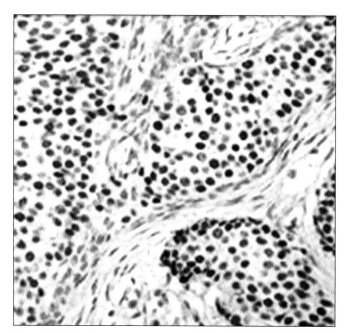

Figure 16.3. This breast cancer section is stained with a monoclonal antibody to estrogen receptor and demonstrates a nuclear staining pattern.

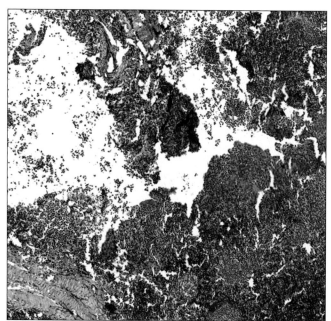

Figure 16.4. Delayed and inadequate fixation, causing complete autolysis of the tissue and loss of antigenicity, is irreversible and can only be prevented by complete fixation before processing.

strongly antigenic tissue is selected, the antibody dilution may be set too high, allowing weakly positive tissue to be falsely reported as negative. As a part of continuous test validation, monitoring of the sensitivity of the antibody is required. Weakly staining tissues will show loss of sensitivity due to aging antibodies more readily than strongly antigenic tissues.

Internal controls are present in some but not all tissues. Examples include estrogen-receptor–positive duct epithelial cells in nonneoplastic breast tissue and S100-positive nerve cells or intraepidermal melanocytes in nonneoplastic skin. The tissue block selected for staining should include both tumor and normal tissue to increase the likelihood that internal controls are present. Internal controls are especially valuable when the fixation of the control tissue and the patient tissue are different.

What Should Be Seen in a Good Immunohistochemical Stain

Each antibody has a specific staining pattern. Information on the expected staining results for each clone is outlined in the antibody specification sheet provided by the vendor. Regardless of the methodology used, all IHC stains should be evaluated using the same criteria. There should be strong, crisp staining of only the target cells and no diffuse staining of the tissue support matrix. The immunoreactivity should show the expected distribution, with staining restricted to the cell membrane (Figure 16.1), cytoplasm (Figure 16.2), nucleus (Figure 16.3), or a combination thereof. There should be no cross-reactivity with, or staining of, nontarget cells. There should be no diffusion of the reaction prod-

uct into surrounding support tissue. There should be no nonspecific staining resulting from endogenous biotin or enzymes such as peroxidase. The counterstain should complement the IHC staining, providing a contrast to the target cells but not masking the delicate staining.

Problems Encountered With Immunohistochemical Stains

PROBLEM: Absence of Staining or Weak Staining of Patient Tissue, With Adequately Stained Positive Control

APPEARANCE: Poorly fixed and processed tissues exhibit uneven or weak staining across the section, combined with intense, dark counterstain (Figure 16.4).

CAUSES:

- Loss of antigenicity was caused by delayed (putrefaction), inadequate (autolysis), or extended (increased numbers of methylene bridges) fixation of the patient tissue.

- The patient tissue was fixed using a method that is different from that used for the control tissue.

- Patient tissue sections were allowed to dry after heat retrieval.

SOLUTIONS:

- Repeat the procedure using a different tissue block that is better fixed or fixed using the same fixative as the control, if available.

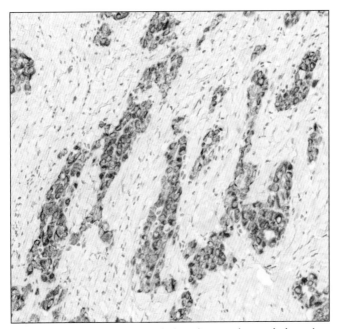

Figure 16.5. The dilution of the antibody in this example is too high, resulting in a low concentration of antibody and poor staining. Compare this image to the well-stained section in Figure 16.2. Overdilution of the antibody can be prevented by validating the antibody using a dilution panel based on the manufacturer's recommended dilution.

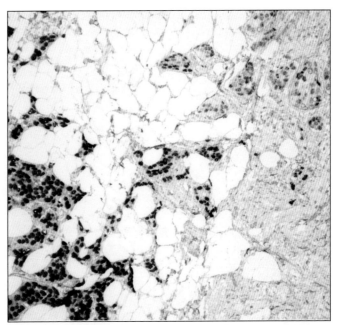

Figure 16.6. Formalin-based fixatives penetrate the tissue at a relatively slow rate, allowing incompletely fixed tissue sections to be postfixed with alcohol on the tissue processor, resulting in different staining intensities, as seen in this breast carcinoma section that is stained for estrogen receptor. Preparation of thin well-fixed blocks is the best way to avoid this phenomenon.

- Repeat the procedure using a more aggressive epitope retrieval protocol (eg, high-pH buffer) to assist with exposure of the target epitopes on the patient's tissue.
- Once deparaffinized, ensure that slides remain wet throughout entire protocol.

PROBLEM: Weak Staining or Absence of Staining, With Weakly Stained Known Positive Control

APPEARANCE: Target cells in the control section display light and uneven detection color (Figure 16.5).

CAUSES:
- The concentration of primary antibody is incorrect.
- There is loss of immunoreactivity due to aging of the stock antibody solution.

SOLUTIONS:
- Re-titer the primary antibody using at least three consecutive dilutions and repeat the validation process on control tissues. Antibodies of the same clone can show different levels of immunoreactivity from lot to lot; therefore, before use, each new lot must be validated using a series of control tissue with known immunoreactivity.

- Repeat, using freshly prepared antibody at the previously determined dilution. Laboratory errors or use of uncalibrated pipettes can result in inaccurate dilutions.
- Repeat, using a more aggressive epitope retrieval protocol (eg, high-pH buffer) to expose the target epitopes.

PROBLEM: No Staining of the Patient or Control Tissues

APPEARANCE: Target cells in the patient and control sections display no detection color (color dependent on the detection reagent used), only color from the counterstain.

CAUSES:
- Primary antibody was not applied, or the wrong primary antibody was applied.
- An incorrect protocol was followed.
- Reagents are expired.

SOLUTIONS:
- Repeat, ensuring that a sufficient quantity of the correct antibody is applied (manual or automated).

- Repeat, after confirming that the correct protocol is being applied and that steps or reagents are not missed or exchanged.
- Repeat, using fresh reagents. Quality management procedures must be in place to ensure outdated reagents are never used.

PROBLEM: Uneven Staining of Patient Tissue

APPEARANCE: The intensity of the staining of the target cells changes across the tissue section (Figure 16.6).

CAUSE:

- There is inadequate primary fixation in formalin, leading to secondary alcohol fixation of parts of the tissue block during processing.

SOLUTIONS:

- Repeat, using a different tissue block with better fixation and processing, if available.
- Repeat, using different epitope retrieval protocols.

PROBLEM: Diffuse Nonspecific Staining of Patient Tissue, With Adequate Positive Control

APPEARANCE: The support matrix surrounding the target cells is staining with the detection reagents, causing background color (Figure 16.7).

CAUSES:

- There was delayed or inadequate fixation of the patient tissue.
- Degenerating cells or necrotic tissue is being evaluated.
- There is nonimmunological binding of detection reagents caused by pseudoperoxidase activity (high concentration of erythrocytes), endogenous peroxidase (seen predominantly in hematopoietic tissue or tissue with hemorrhage), or endogenous biotin.

SOLUTIONS:

- Fix patient tissue using a standardized protocol.
- Repeat, using a different tissue block, if available.
- Repeat, using a less vigorous epitope retrieval protocol (Figure 16.8), because over-retrieval can expose nontarget epitopes.
- Incorporate pretreatment steps to block endogenous peroxidase and biotin in patient tissues.

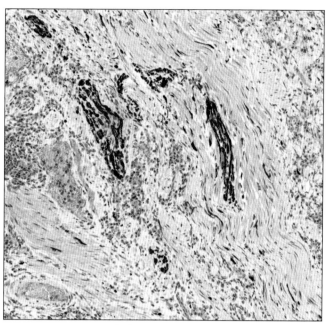

Figure 16.7. Aggressive, high-pH, heat-induced epitope retrieval was used, resulting in nonspecific background staining from the exposure of nontarget epitopes. Testing multiple retrieval methods during the antibody validation process will identify the best retrieval method for specific antibodies.

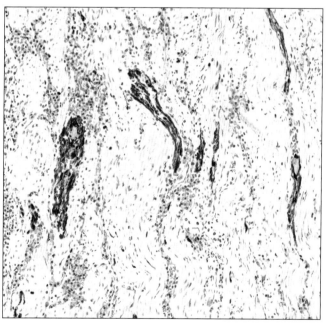

Figure 16.8. Enzyme retrieval used on a section from the same tissue block as in Figure 16.7, with the same antibody concentration, results in only the target cells staining and a clean background.

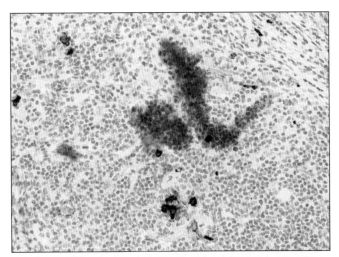

Figure 16.9. Detection system reagents may become trapped in areas of tissue detachment, resulting in false-positive staining. This artifact can be avoided by using a slide adhesive and drying sections appropriately to ensure secure tissue attachment to the slide.

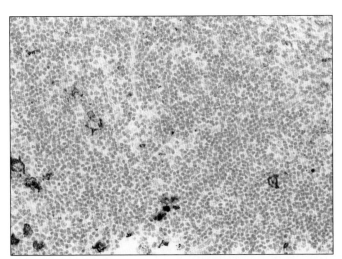

Figure 16.10. Antibody to CD15 is used to demonstrate Reed-Sternberg cells, the larger cells in this image. As part of the normal staining pattern, granulocytes also stain; this pattern is not considered false-positive staining.

PROBLEM: Nonspecific Staining of the Patient and Control Tissues

APPEARANCE: The support matrix surrounding the target cells is staining with the detection reagents, causing background color or limited, defined areas of nonspecific staining (Figure 16. 9).

CAUSES:

- There is microbial or chemical contamination of the reagents.
- Normal serum used for blocking is from the same species as the secondary antibody.
- Detection substrate is trapped between the tissue and the slide.

SOLUTIONS:

- Always dilute, dispense, and store primary antibodies and reagents according to manufacturer's instructions.
- Ensure equipment used to make and store all reagents is clean—or sterile, if required. Rinse well with distilled water to remove detergents used for cleaning. Thoroughly dry glassware before use.
- Ensure that the blocking serum is from the same species and is at the same protein concentration as the primary antibody.
- Repeat with sections that do not have wrinkles or air bubbles under the section where chromagen from the detection kit can become trapped.
- Use a slide with a strong adhesive, such as silane (aminopropyltriethoxysilane), to ensure section attachment to the slide.

PROBLEM: False-Positive Staining of Nontarget Cells

APPEARANCE: Cells that are not associated with the tumor are displaying detection color; often the staining pattern in nontarget cells is different from that of the target cells (Figure 16.10).

CAUSE:

- There is cross-reactivity of the antibody with tissue cellular components.

SOLUTIONS:

- Polyclonal antibodies can be affinity purified via a process that removes the "nonspecific" immunoglobulin.
- Use a monoclonal antibody, if available. Monoclonal antibodies are generated using hybridoma technology, which yields clones of antibody-producing cells, such that each clone produces an antibody directed against a single, target-specific epitope.
- Compare the IHC slide to the corresponding hematoxylin-and-eosin slide and identify tumor versus nontumor cells to ensure the target cells are being evaluated.

PROBLEM: Nonspecific Staining of Patient Tissue, With Overstained Positive Control and Overstained Specific Target Cells in Patient Tissue

APPEARANCE: Staining pattern of the target cells is very intense, often obscuring cellular details; or the support matrix surrounding the target cells is staining with the detection reagents, causing background color (Figure 16.11).

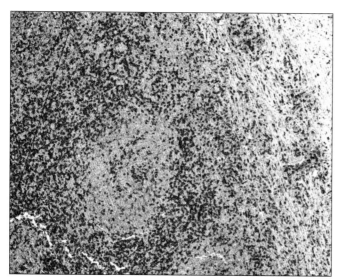

Figure 16.11. Failure to use the correct dilution of the antibody can result in overstaining of the target cells and staining of the supporting tissue matrix. All neat-sera antibodies must be validated using a series of dilutions to establish the correct dilution before use on patient tissues.

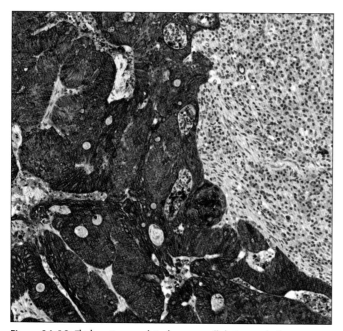

Figure 16.12. Thick sections result in the target cells being too dark to interpret. Also, the higher concentration of counterstain obscures details. Establish a tissue section thickness that will be used for all IHC control and patient slides. Validation against a standardized section will ensure consistent staining quality.

CAUSES:

- Concentration of the primary antibody is too strong.
- Tissue sections are too thick (Figure 16.12).

SOLUTIONS:

- Check dilution of antibody and repeat the procedure using freshly prepared antibody. Laboratory errors or

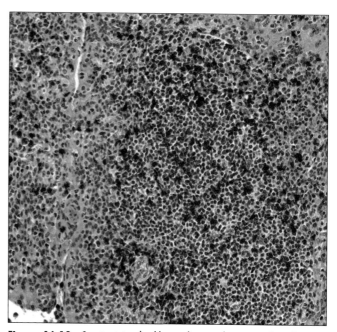

Figure 16.13. Counterstain should complement the immunohistochemistry staining and provide enough definition to evaluate tissue morphology, but not obscure details. The counterstain can be adjusted by altering concentration of the stain or reducing staining time.

use of uncalibrated pipettes can result in inaccurate dilutions.

- Re-titer primary antibody using at least three consecutive dilutions, and repeat validation process on control tissues. Antibodies of the same clone can change concentration from lot to lot; each new lot requires validation before use.

- Cut all sections at the same thickness as the section used to validate antibody dilution. Thick sections can result in the localization of more antibody and result in overstaining.

PROBLEM: Counterstain Masks Delicate Antibody-Specific Staining

APPEARANCE: All cells have an intense blue color from the hematoxylin counterstain (Figure 16.13).

CAUSES:

- Staining time for counterstain is too long.
- Concentration of the counterstain is too strong.

SOLUTION:

- Decrease staining time in hematoxylin or use a weaker solution of hematoxylin.

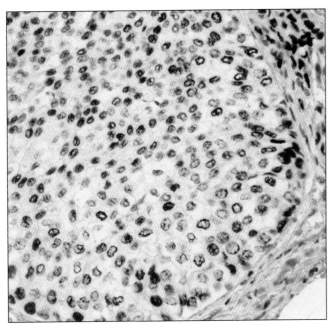

Figure 16.14. If precut control slides are not dried or stored at an appropriate temperature, the result will be a continued loss of antigenicity as storage continues. Note the loss of nuclear stain in this section of breast cancer; this tumor was initially intensely positive for estrogen receptor. Use the antibody vendor's guidelines to establish a protocol for how control slides should be cut and stored.

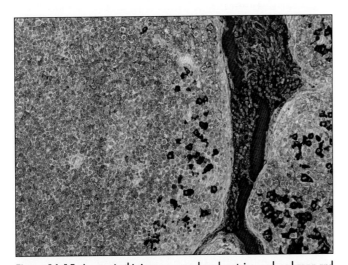

Figure 16.15. As seen in this image, serum-based proteins, such as kappa and lambda (immunoglobulin light chains), may leak from the cell and react with the antibody outside the cell membrane.

PROBLEM: Decreasing Intensity of Known Control Staining Over a Time Period

APPEARANCE: Stained target cells in the most recently stained control section appear lighter when compared with the target cells in the identical control section originally stained to validate the control tissue block. Target cells appear pale or faded (Figure 16.14).

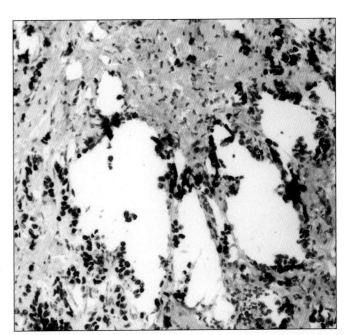

Figure 16.16. Severe tissue detachment affects the tissue morphology and results in the inability to interpret the stain. Use of well-fixed tissue sections attached to charged slides can assist in avoiding tissue loss.

CAUSES:

- Control tissue has aged.
- Precut control was not stored at correct temperature.

SOLUTIONS:

- Cut the control section immediately before use.
- Do not dry control slides at high temperature or for extended time.

PROBLEM: Diffusion of Detection Product

APPEARANCE: Amorphous masses of detection color appear outside the target cells (Figure 16.15).

CAUSE:

- Serum-based proteins can diffuse from the cell and react with the detection reagent outside the cell.

SOLUTION:

- Place tissue into fixative as soon as possible after removal from the patient.

PROBLEM: Tissue Detachment

APPEARANCE: The overall appearance of the tissue section is ragged, and the tissue morphology is destroyed (Figure 16.16).

CAUSES:

- The epitope retrieval step was excessively vigorous.
- The tissue was poorly fixed or poorly processed, or both.

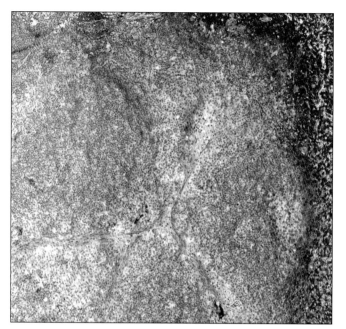

Figure 16.17. Automation has produced a great improvement in immunohisto-chemistry staining but also brings a new set of artifacts to be identified, such as uneven application of the detection reagents. Cleaning and regular maintenance of all instrumentation is essential to ensure consistent operation.

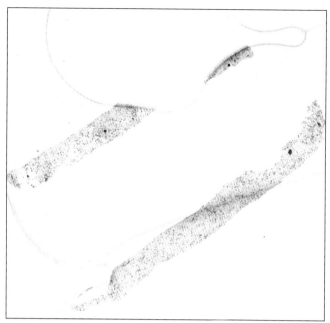

Figure 16.19. Areas where paraffin is not removed will not stain with immuno-histochemistry techniques or counterstain. Use a procedure to dry slides that will avoid pooling of large amounts of paraffin on the slide when cold.

- Use a slide with a strong adhesive, such as amino-propyltriethoxysilane.

PROBLEM: Uneven Deposition of Detection Reagent

APPEARANCE: Areas of the tumor or target cells are not stained with the detection reagent; often there is a definite line between stained and nonstained areas. In contrast, all areas are counterstained with hematoxylin (Figures 16.17 and 16.18).

CAUSE:

- Incomplete mixing or uneven application of detection reagent by automated instrumentation.

SOLUTIONS:

- Maintain all automated equipment as per manufac-turers' guidelines.
- Follow manufacturers' operating instructions.
- Allow only fully trained staff to operate equipment.

PROBLEM: Failure of Portions of Section to Stain With Antibody or Counterstain

APPEARANCE: Areas of the tumor or target cells appear as opaque white, having no color from the detec-tion reagent or counterstain (Figure 16.19).

CAUSE:

- Removal of paraffin is incomplete.

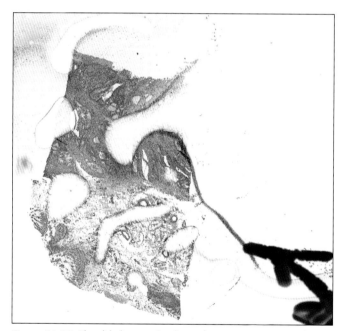

Figure 16.18. This slide became dry during the staining process, resulting in uneven application of the detection reagents. Visual inspection of the stainer and consumable reagents before use is essential to avoid operational failures.

SOLUTIONS:

- Repeat, using a less vigorous epitope retrieval proto-col, such as a weaker enzyme concentration or less time in hot retrieval fluids.
- Increase slide-drying time.

SOLUTIONS:

- Ensure sections are completely covered with dewaxing reagents.
- Maintain all automated equipment as per manufacturers' guidelines.
- Follow manufacturers' operating instructions.
- Allow only fully trained staff to operate equipment.

Bibliography

College of American Pathologists (CAP) Certification Program for Immunohistochemistry. Northfield, Ill: College of American Pathologists; 2007: 41-48.

Dapson R, Feldman AT, Wolfe D. *Lessons in Immunohistochemistry.* Battle Creek, MI: Anatech Ltd; 2005.

Key M, et al. *Handbook of Immunochemical Staining Methods.* 4th ed. California: Dako Cytomation; 2006.

Ladik CL, White CL. Immunohistochemistry quality control. In: Bancroft J, Gamble M, eds. *Theory and Practice of Histological Techniques.* 6th ed. New York, NY: Churchill Livingstone; 2008: 473-491.

Leong AS-Y, Cooper K, Leong FJW-M. *Manual of Diagnostic Antibodies for Immunohistology.* 2nd ed. London, England: Greenwich Medical Media; 2003.

Nadji M, Morales A. *Immunoperoxidase Techniques: A Practical Approach to Tumor Diagnosis.* Chicago, IL: American Society of Clinical Pathologists; 1986.

Quality Assurance for Immunocytochemistry. Approved Guideline. Wayne, PA: NCCLS (now Clinical and Laboratory Standards Institute [CLSI]); 1999. Document MM4-A.

Acidophilic: A basic (cationic, positively charged) tissue component that attracts an acidic (anionic, negatively charged) dye. The most commonly used acidic dye is eosin, which stains acidophilic structures red and is the source of the related term eosinophilic.

Additive: A substance that adds on to, or combines with, another substance. This occurs during the process of tissue fixation when fixatives add on to tissue proteins, altering and stabilizing them in the process.

Amphoterism: The property of some compounds in solution to exhibit either positive or negative charges, depending on the pH of the solution.

Anionic: A negatively charged dye or tissue component, sometimes referred to as acidic, that binds to a cationic dye or tissue component.

Argentaffin: A reaction in which tissue substances have both the ability to bind or be impregnated with silver ions and reduce the silver to its visible metallic form.

Argyrophilic: The ability to bind or be impregnated with silver ions; a reducing agent is required to reduce the silver ions to a visible metallic end product.

Artifact: A substance or structure that is not normally present but that has been produced by some external force. Substances such as formalin and mercury pigments and structures such as knife lines and air bubbles are examples.

Autolysis: Digestion or destruction of tissue or cells by enzymes present in the tissue.

Basophilic: An acidic (anionic, negatively charged) tissue component that attracts a basic (cationic, positively charged) dye. The most commonly used basic dye is hematoxylin. In hematoxylin-and-eosin (H&E)–stained sections, basophilic structures are usually those that contain nucleic acid, such as the cell nucleus and ribosomes.

Beading: Granular deposition of silver on or around the tissue elements.

Birefringence: The splitting of a single light wave into two waves that are reflected in different directions; this is also known as anisotropism and double refraction.

Cationic: A positively charged dye or tissue component, sometimes referred to as basic, that binds to an anionic dye or tissue component.

Chromatin: A complex of nucleic acids and proteins, primarily histones, in the cell nucleus that stains readily with basic dyes and condenses to form chromosomes during cell division. In light microscopy, this term refers to the primary stainable substance in the nucleus.

Chatter: Parallel defects in tissue sections resembling Venetian blinds.

Clearance angle: The angle formed between the cutting facet of the blade and the paraffin block as the blade is tilted.

Clearing: The removal of the dehydrating solution from tissues in preparation for either paraffin infiltration (processing) or coverslipping (staining).

Counterstain: A stain that will give contrast to the tissue elements being demonstrated by the principal stain. A counterstain should enhance or help visualize secondary tissue elements, never masking the structures of primary interest in the tissue.

Dehydration: The removal of free water from tissues.

Denaturation: Changing the nature or shape of large molecules. Fixatives denature proteins by changing liquid cellular contents into insoluble substances; this ensures that those substances are not lost during the subsequent processing steps.

Deparaffinization: The first step in any histologic staining method, through which the paraffin in the tissue section is removed by xylene (or xylene substitute) and is replaced with water.

Differentiation: Decolorization, or the removal of excess color from tissue. This is done with acidic or basic solutions, excess mordant, or oxidizers. Proper differentiation allows tissue structures to be distinguished from one another by differing color or staining intensity.

Dye: A molecule that possesses specific chemical groupings in its molecular structure that impart color as well as the ability to form chemical bonds with tissues.

Embedding: Enclosing the tissue in a medium that will solidify and allow the cutting of thin sections.

Fixation: The stabilization of proteins that is undertaken to preserve tissue structures and prevent autolysis.

Floaters: Foreign material picked up from the flotation bath on a tissue section. This can be squamous cells or debris from either the current tissue being sectioned or a previous tissue.

Hydrophilic: The physical property of a molecule that can transiently bond with water through hydrogen bonds.

Hydrophobic: The physical property of a molecule that is repelled from a mass of water.

Impregnation: Deposition of salts of gold or silver on or around, but not in, the tissue components to be demonstrated.

Isoelectric point: The pH at which an amphoteric substance in solution will possess no net charge; the number of positive and negative charges is equal.

Metachromasia: A characteristic of some dyes to exhibit more than one color when bound to tissue structures that allow the bound dye molecules to be in such close proximity to each other that they are able to interact in such a manner as to elicit a different color.

Micrometer: The dial on a microtome that allows one to change the thickness at which sections are cut.

Mirroring: The breakdown of methenamine silver at temperatures in excess of 50°C, resulting in the formation of gray metallic precipitate on the inside of the stain vessel or on the slide.

Mordant: A reagent that links the stain, or dye molecules, to tissue. Aluminum is the mordant in hematoxylin solutions used in the routine hematoxylin and eosin (H&E) stain, and iron is the mordant in Verhoeff hematoxylin.

Oxidation: A chemical reaction in which molecules combine with oxygen or there is loss of electrons (and/or hydrogen atoms).

Progressive staining: Staining to the desired intensity and stopping the stain. No differentiation step is used. Most counterstains are used progressively.

Reduction: A chemical reaction in which there is loss of oxygen atoms or the gain of electrons/hydrogen atoms by the molecules.

Regressive staining: Overstaining and then removing the excess stain (differentiation) by either an acid or base, excess mordant, or oxidizers until the desired tissue component contrasts sharply with the background. The Verhoeff elastic stain is an example of regressive staining that is differentiated with excess mordant.

Saturated: A solution that contains an amount of ionized salt equal to its maximum solubility.

Sensitization: An impregnation technique in which a metal salt (silver nitrate, uranyl nitrate) forms a metallic organic compound with the tissue.

Supersaturated: A solution that contains more of the dissolved material than could be dissolved by the solvent under normal circumstances; typically, supersaturated solutions are achieved with heating.

Toning: The deposition of gold at the site of reduced (metallic) silver. The silver impregnation is partially converted to a gold impregnation by treatment with gold chloride.

Index

absolute ethanol, 79
acid alcohol, 57
acid-fast bacilli (AFB), 59
acid-fast bacteria, 57-58
acquired immune deficiency syndrome (AIDS), 57, 86
additive fixatives, 139
AIDS-associated systemic bacterial infection, 57
Alcian blue stain, 86, 125, 133
    problems encountered with, 128-130
Alcian yellow-toluidine blue (AY-TB) technique, 67
alcohol patterns, 1
alcoholic eosin, 36
alcoholic fixatives, 1-2
aldehyde fuchsin, 109, 110, 114-115
alum hematoxylins, 35, 96
ammoniacal silver reaction, 103
ammonium hydroxide, 103
amylase, 79
amyloid, 133-137
    Alcian blue stain, 133
    birefringence, 133, 134
    Congo red stain, 133-134
        good, 134
        Puchtler method, 134
    controls, 134
    fluorochrome thioflavin T stain, 133
    periodic acid-Schiff stain, 133
    problems encountered with the Congo red stain
        incorrect color of birefringence, 136
        nonspecific staining, 135-136
        precipitate on tissue, 137
        weakly stained tissues, 135
    Sirius red stain, 133
amyloidosis, 133
anionic dyes, 95-96
antibody selection and use, 139
antigen retrieval, 139-140
aqueous fixatives, 1
artifact, ice crystal (freeze), 28
artifacts, in microtomy, 15, 16
auramine-rhodamine method, 58

bacteria. *See also* Gram stain; *Helicobacter pylori;* mycobacteria; spirochetes
    acid-fast, 57-58, 59
    cell wall structure, 49
    classification of, 51
    Gram stain, 49-56
    inflammation from, 49
    stains for, 49

basement membrane (BM), 117-123
    components, 117
    controls, 117
    glomerular basement membrane (GBM), 117
    good stain for, 118
    periodic acid-methenamine silver (PAMS) method, 117
    periodic acid-Schiff (PAS) method, 117
    problems encountered in the methenamine silver reaction
        determining the end point, 118-119
        difficulty keeping tissue section on slide, 120
        nonspecific staining of tissue elements, or precipitate on tissue, or both, 119
        sections overtoned in gold chloride, 121
        uneven staining, 120-121
    problems encountered in the periodic acid-Schiff reaction
        nonspecific background staining, 122
        reaction not as bright as expected; GBMs not stained adequately, 121-122
        Schiff reaction masked by counterstain, 122-123
B5, 96
Biebrich scarlet stain, 109
birefringence, 133, 134-136
blue halo effect, 2
bone dust, 11
Bouin solution, 96
Brown and Brenn (B&B) procedure, 50
Brown-Hopps (B&H) procedure, 50
bubbles, from microtomy, 24-25

calcium salts, 79
carbolfuchsin stains, 49, 57. *See also* fuchsin
cell shrinkage, 7
chatter, microscopic, 6, 15, 20
chromic acid, 86, 117
Chromotrope 2R, 96
citrate, 140
coagulating fixatives, 139
College of American Pathologists (CAP), 2, 15, 37
colloidal iron stain, 86
controls
    for basement membrane stains, 117
    for elastin stains, 110-111
    for frozen sections, 31
    for fungi, 87
    for Gram stains, 52
    for H&E stains, 36
    for *Helicobacter pylori,* 69
    for immunohistochemical stains, 140-141
    for mucin stains, 126
    for mycobacteria, 59